I0085880

A Skeptic's Journey
through the
Yoga Experience

A Skeptic's Journey through the Yoga Experience

by
Earl Ofari Hutchinson

MID|DLE
PASS|AGE
P R E S S

A Skeptic's Journey through the Yoga Experience

Copyright © 2017 Earl Ofari Hutchinson
All rights reserved including the right of reproduction in whole or in part in any form.

Printed in the United States

Published by
Middle Passage Press
5517 Secrest Drive
Los Angeles, California 90043

Photographs by Angela Hoffman
Book designed by Alan Bell

Publisher's Cataloging-in-Publication data

Names: Hutchinson, Earl Ofari, author.
Title: A Skeptic's journey through the yoga experience / Earl Ofari Hutchinson.
Description: Includes bibliographical references and index. | Los Angeles, CA: Middle Passage Press: 2017
Identifiers: ISBN 978057819408-0
Subjects: LCSH Yoga. | Hatha yoga—United States—History. | BISAC HEALTH & FITNESS / Yoga
Classification: LCC RA781.7 .H88 2017 | DDC 613.7/046—dc23

LCCN: 2017915018

To Melinda Smith
who taught me the true meaning of yoga
and much more
and to seniors who believe that wellness
begins not ends at 60

Table of Contents

A Skeptic's Journey
through the
Yoga Experience

Introduction

I must first make a full disclosure. My first experience with yoga was an absolute disaster. It was spring, 2009. I decided that I needed to take an exercise class to improve my muscle and joint flexibility. As a long-time distance runner, flexibility, or the lack thereof, was a chronic problem for me. This comes with the runner's turf, especially for male runners.

I searched the course catalogue of a nearby college for such a class. The course that caught my eye was beginning yoga. It was the only PE class at a time and day that fit my work schedule. I signed up for it. But I felt trepidation and unease. I quickly realized why. I carried a train station full of baggage about what yoga was, and who yoga appealed to. Put bluntly, I thought it was too white, too feminine, too exotic, too taxing, and too removed from my life. The storehouse of negatives I brought to yoga did not bode well. In fact, it almost guaranteed that the negatives would inevitably become a self-fulfilling prophecy.

It didn't take long. The first day of class, I was only one of two men in the class of about 20. The instructor, though pleasant enough, quickly put us though a first day regimen of deep leg lifts, splits, leg raises, and other poses that seemed to me way too taxing. They were simply way beyond my level of flexibility. I lasted all of two sessions in the class. This seemed to confirm the doubts and the prior ingrained negative conception I had about the usefulness of yoga.

* * * * *

For the next four years, yoga was as far from my mind as the distance between the sun and moon. The infrequent occasions someone would mention that they were in a yoga class, I would instantly tune out. Then something happened that stood the negative thoughts and abbreviated experience I had with yoga on its head. Flexibility remained a chronic problem

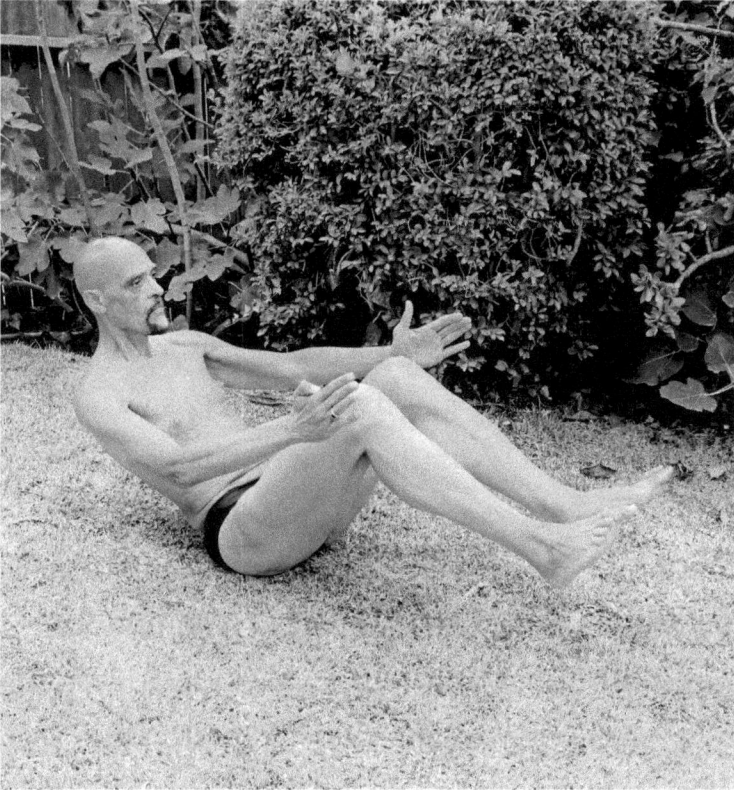

Nauv Asana (Boat Pose)

due to my running. So, I thought, maybe, just maybe, I'd take another crack at taking a class to improve my flexibility. Again, the only class available at the nearby college that fit my tight work schedule I was on was, of course, yoga.

I couldn't totally shake the bad experience I had with the yoga class four years earlier from my mind. However, the time, and the day the class was offered was convenient. With the same trepidation and deep reluctance as before, I signed up. A voice, though, still whispered in my head, "take a quick look in, probably find the same excuses as before, and then make a quick exit."

When I arrived at the class, the gender ratio hadn't changed much. There were a handful of guys there, and the rest of the class of about thirty were women. I discretely found a spot at the rear of the class, near the back door. My body leaned toward the exit.

I had barely found a spot to sit, when the instructor, Melinda Smith, spied me. In a soft, pleasant voice she said, "There's a spot over here, why don't you move closer in." There was something reassuring in her voice that immediately put me at ease. I moved in closer and listened as she outlined what the class entailed. She made it clear that no one was in competition with anyone else in the class. You worked through the poses and movements at your own pace.

She continually noted that everybody is different, and that the point of yoga is to relax, enjoy it, and find your own level of physical and mental comfort. Her words were instantly transformative. This was an instructor, I felt, who truly cared about the students, the practice of yoga, and wanted others to feel the same about it. Her words and admonition about the purpose and practice of yoga made me feel not just as another student in another class, but part of a real life affirming experience.

* * * * *

This was the start of a journey, a journey that for the next five years would take me through many facets of the yoga experience. In *A Skeptic's Journey through the Yoga Experience,* I will take the reader through my excursion through the yoga experience. I look at the history, the myths, the controversies, the practice, the philosophy, the growth, commercialism of, and impact of yoga. I also examine the racial and gender conceptions and controversies that confront yoga, as well as the controversy and debate over the physical hazards of yoga to men especially.

Yoga dates back more than 5000 years. So, I emphasize that this is a small primer solely to give a skeptic's impressions of some of the hot button issues and controversies in the yoga world. It in no way pretends to be a comprehensive and definitive study of yoga. There is a library full of books and studies that examine in depth the history, philosophy, and practices of yoga, as well as the many schools of yoga.

Also, at different periods during my practice of, and the courses I have taken in yoga, I have kept a journal noting my feelings, and thoughts about the various poses, movements, and mental and physical changes and benefits of yoga. I intersperse my yoga journal notes throughout *A Skeptic's Journey through the Yoga Experience.* The aim is to personalize the huge impact that yoga has had on my life.

In my small way, with this work, I seek, to pay tribute to the instructors who have given and continue to give generously of their time, energy, patience, and marvelous dedication and devotion to yoga to me. Above all, I want to share the transforming experience I have had with yoga with you.

1
A Walk through Yoga's Past

I had a mental freeze frame for years when I thought of yoga. The image was one of young, slender, athletic looking women going through a variety of gymnastic looking poses, with barely pronounceable, Hindu names. The view was superficial, uniformed, and stereotypical. However, when I enrolled in my second yoga class years later, I quickly found there was more, much more, to yoga than those glamor, superficial commercial shots in magazines ads.

Yoga has a history, a very long and rich history. I vaguely knew that a huge part of that history was its grounding in spiritualism and that its origin was in India and Hinduism. This was only the start. To un-

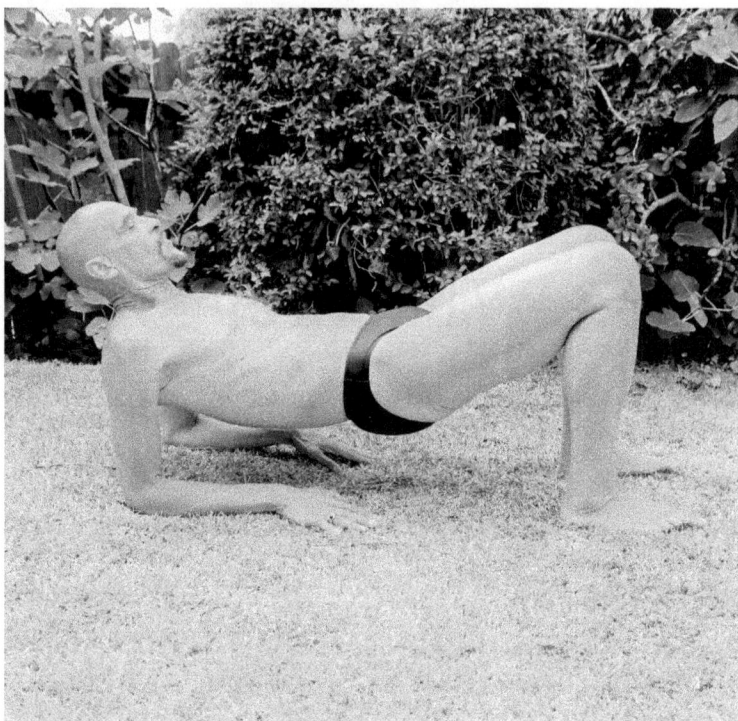

Setu Bandhasana (Bridge Pose)

derstand how yoga originated and its true purpose, I had to familiarize myself with the jargon of yoga. The starting point was the word itself. Yoga is a Sanskrit word. Sanskrit is the very oldest of old languages of India. Yoga literally means to unite an individual with their consciousness and awareness of the world. This is just vague and expansive enough to permit individuals to give free reign to just how they see and perceive the world around them. And how their thoughts and actions are deeply influenced by that awareness. It's strictly an individual thing.

The operative word I learned in yoga is the *Veda*. This is foundational to a knowledge and appreciation of the principles and practices and end goal of yoga. *Veda,* in the Oxford Dictionary, is defined as the most ancient Hindu scriptures, written in early Sanskrit and containing hymns, philosophy, and guidance on ritual for the priests of the Vedic religion. It is believed to have been directly revealed to seers among the early Aryans in India, and preserved by oral tradition. The four chief collections are the *Rig Veda, Sama Veda, Yajur Veda,* and *Atharva Veda.*

I next discovered this was just the tip of the yoga

iceberg. There are sub *Vedas* and each of these has a hierarchy of meaning and knowledge with labels such as *upangas,* and the *upangas* have their subs too. They all have Sanskrit names and meanings. This wouldn't be complete without a book that brought this all together into some kind of working order. The book is the *Rigveda* which was around thousands of years before the Bible was written. That gives it the distinction of being the oldest book of sacred verses in existence.

This is my third semester in Melinda Smith's yoga class. The first semester was an eye opening, pure learning experience about yoga. I approached it with anxiety. My two great fears were my age, and muscular inflexibility. Namely, that I might not be able to keep up with the movements required, and that they were for younger persons. That fear dissipated quickly. It dissipated partly through the structure, patience, and insight of the instructor, and partly through my willingness to challenge my body in ways that I hadn't before. The flexibility concern was over

the stiffness and lack of muscular flexibility from years of running. I overcame that through the willingness to push my body (and mind).

* * * * *

The man who is generally acknowledged to be the one who put the spiritual body to yoga is Maharishi Patanjali. He put a code of practice to the sacred verses. He laid it out in what he called the famed "eight limbs" of yoga that comprise a code of conduct, personal ethics, consciousness of one's self, as well as what and how to focus the mind. The twin pillars of yoga, and are the ones that are the best known and popular, and mark the yoga practice, are the poses, or postures, and meditation. The poses are called *asanas.* The textbook definition of an asana is a posture in which a practitioner sits. These are the traditional sitting positions or more commonly "yoga positions." They are performed as physical exercises. The pictures of rows of participants in yoga classes and sessions have become standard fare in the promotion of yoga to American.

As with any big, sweeping religion and spiritual practice, it wasn't long before others came along with their own versions and interpretations of what yoga is and how it should be practiced. They also had to have unique names to distinguish one from the other. Here are a few of them: *Gyan yoga, Bhakti yoga, Karma yoga, Hatha yoga, Raj yoga, Mantra yoga, Shiva yoga, Naad yoga, Laya yoga.* Needless to say, there are a lot more of them.

These are just names to most people. But to those who are interested in knowing more about the origins of yoga, the big problem is that most people often don't get much further along in understanding the point of yoga than identifying yoga with those twisting, gymnastic looking physical postures that characterize yoga in the popular mind and culture.

What's missed is that the postures tied to the yoga philosophy are not the end in themselves. They are the means to lead an individual to a higher awareness of his or her self. Skilled yoga instructors constantly talk about the importance of breathing, focus, and clearing the mind of the day-to-day clutter and baggage of worries, problems, and negative thoughts while going through those postures.

There is an entire literature that talks about the

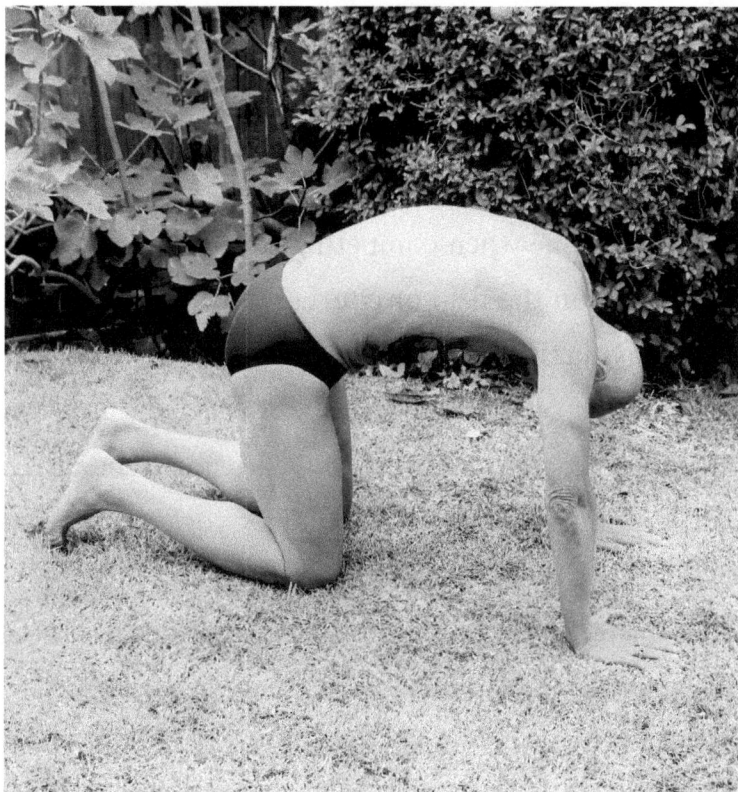

Marjaria Asana (Cat Pose)

importance of getting into the proper "mind set" while doing the varied yoga postures. The idea is to use the postures to induce a calm, relaxed, reflective state of mind and well-being. It's similar to an athlete finding his or her zone when competing to attain their maximum best on the field or court. The difference is that the individual isn't competing with anyone else. Nor is he or she competing with themselves. It's a means to find a peaceful moment of well-being. One of the better known and more popular of yoga practices is *Hatha yoga.*

I heard of *Hatha yoga* long before I started taking yoga classes. I read a book titled *Raja Yoga or Mental Development: A Series of Lessons.* It talked about the asanas. However, it also detailed the Hindu philosophy of life. At the time, they were just words, and had little meaning for me. They reinforced the thought that this was really exotic stuff, best to be put aside for another day or forgotten.

*   *   *   *   *

There was something else at the time that intrigued me and fired my curiosity about yoga. That was just how this foreign, almost alien, practice, had all of sudden become the rage in the U.S.

I thought it was just another one of the fads of the 1960s, immortalized in pop culture by Woodstock, San Francisco's Haight Ashbury District, the love ins, and the counter-culture stuff of the times.

Not so, yoga was introduced to the U.S. in the 19th century. The great philosophical rebels of that era, Ralph Waldo Emerson and Henry David Thoreau were infatuated with Hindu religious verses and practices. Thoreau read the Hindu classics, adopted a spartan diet, that included fasting, and meditated for hours on the great problems of the day. At the close of the century, one of India's leading Swami's made a whirlwind tour of the U.S. to raise money to aid India's impoverished masses.

The Swami stopped off at the World Parliament of Religion in 1893. He brought the house down with his stem winding speeches on Hindu philosophy, religion, and practices. One of which was the practice of yoga. Apart from a few ascetics, outlier spiritualists, herbalists, naturopaths, assorted mystics, and just plain quacks, for the most part, yoga remained an obscure, esoteric and largely forgotten practice for the next six decades. That changed in the 1960s when several of India's leading Swamis, riding the crest of the counter culture boom of the day, trekked to this country. They drew wildly adoring crowds to their talks, lectures, mass meditation, yoga posture sessions and demonstrations throughout the country.

* * * * *

Some stayed around for extended periods to set up a string of retreats and "spiritual centers" throughout the country. For a hefty fee, the curious, and the spiritual wisdom seekers could hang their hats for days on end at them sitting in rapt attention listening to assorted Swami's and yoga teachers and practitioners dispense their pearls of philosophical wisdom and then be taken through the ropes on yoga principles and practices.

Yoga had finally come out of the shadows in the 1960s and become a respected and much practiced movement to promote mental and spiritual well-being. Its added by-product was that it could be a means to enhance one's muscle flexibility and muscle tone. The importance of the health benefit can't be over stated.

Yoga would not have drawn me to it if there were no promise of it helping wring the stiffness out of my aging muscles and joints. Many others who have written and discussed their motivation for taking up yoga have said the same. They primarily see yoga as a good physical workout and a way to improve their flexibility.

In fact, in the half century since yoga exploded on the scene in the U.S. it has totally undergone a transformation. It is regarded as one of the best natural therapies. Some go further and ascribe to it almost mystical powers to cure almost all physical and emotional ills and woes.

Many yoga enthusiasts endlessly cite the passage in the *Bhagavad Gita,* where Lord Krishna says, "Samatvam Yoga Uchyate"—equanimity in the mind is a sign of yoga. The claim is that the practice can keep one "centered" in any and every adverse situation. Yoga pros are careful not to claim that yoga is the passport to the happy life. However, the notion that it can dangles heavily in the air whenever yoga enthusiasts cite the virtues of yoga.

The claim of the power to heal physical and emotional ailments has always been a major fascination and selling point of yoga. Yet, this is not what made the sale for me. The years of studying and practicing it, has been its own reward for me. In that sense, I can say, that yoga has fulfilled its promise of providing moments of calm and inner peace in troubling situations. Equally important, it has done what brought me to it initially, and that's restore a degree of flexibility to the muscles in the old body.

2

Take a Yoga Break

I have heard it said so often that I can virtually cite it by rote in my sleep. The "it" is that yoga is one of human kind's great stress relievers. You have a bad day at school or the office; take a yoga break. You have an argument with your wife, husband, significant other, or anyone else; take a yoga break. You have chronic worries over bills, personal relations, or physical ailments; take a yoga break. Clearly, for the most exuberant yoga devotee, yoga is as close to the magic pill for every sort of human ailment one can imagine.

The question of just what yoga can and can't do for you has been bandied about so often by legions of medical professionals, scientists, and researchers that it has become a common place in the literature of medical treatments. In fact, yoga is well on its way to being one of the most studied alternative practices around. One researcher who crunched the numbers found that the number of studies of what yoga can do for the mind and body jumped by a factor of 10 in the number of yoga-related scientific papers per year since the late 1990's. In 2013, there were 74 studies published which set a pace for 380 yoga-related studies that year. There has been no drop off in years after in the number of articles that debate the pros and cons of yoga.

Just what have all the experts made of these studies? First, their conclusions are based almost exclusively on interviews and responses of subjects asked to rate their health and fitness and wellness before, during, and after a yoga session. In other words, their findings are mostly anecdotal. There is no precise way to quantify whether a group of subjects who practice yoga and who report high blood pressure have experienced a consistent drop in their blood pressure, let alone prove there is a direct cause and effect tie to yoga. This requires a control group, double blind studies, and a longitudinal study to pin down an answer.

Still, the general consensus among many observers who have no product to sell, axe to grind, or who aren't true believers in the practice, is that yoga can have some benefit for some ailments, such as to help relieve anxiety, insomnia, depression, and back pain. It has also been found to help lower heart rate and blood pressure. For many person's, it has proven helpful in improving strength, flexibility and general fitness. Again, this was the selling point for me, and from studies, this has been the motivator for many Americans to try yoga.

* * * * *

The operative word, though I, and most medical experts use, is "help." The word doctors who see benefits to alternative treatments use when the subject of alternative treatments for sickness and conditions arises is "complementary." This means that it's something that can be used in conjunction with standard medical treatment, not before, and certainly not as a replacement for treatment.

An individual who is chronically stressed out, or suffers anxiety attacks, can't simply do a down dog pose, breathe ten times, meditate for five minutes, and expect that the stress or anxiety will instantly disappear like a Houdini magic act. There's a little thing called "cause"; namely what are the underlying issues that cause the stress in the first place. To find lasting relief from these symptoms, requires intense counseling and therapy to get to their root causes.

Someone who suffers a serious heart condition, diabetes, or chronic back pain, would not suddenly toss away their medication, pain pills, cancel their doctor's appointments, and rush to a yoga session for a quick cure. There's also the question of individual differences. That is how individuals perceive pain and deal with it. This is the mindset that yoga practitioners endlessly talk about as the major pay-off from yoga. There is much truth to the adage how we think is how we feel. There is extensive literature that examines the connection between how individuals perceive and react to pain and physical and emotional discomfort. Many do find a direct connect between mental well-being, and the ability to minimize pain. Yoga is often

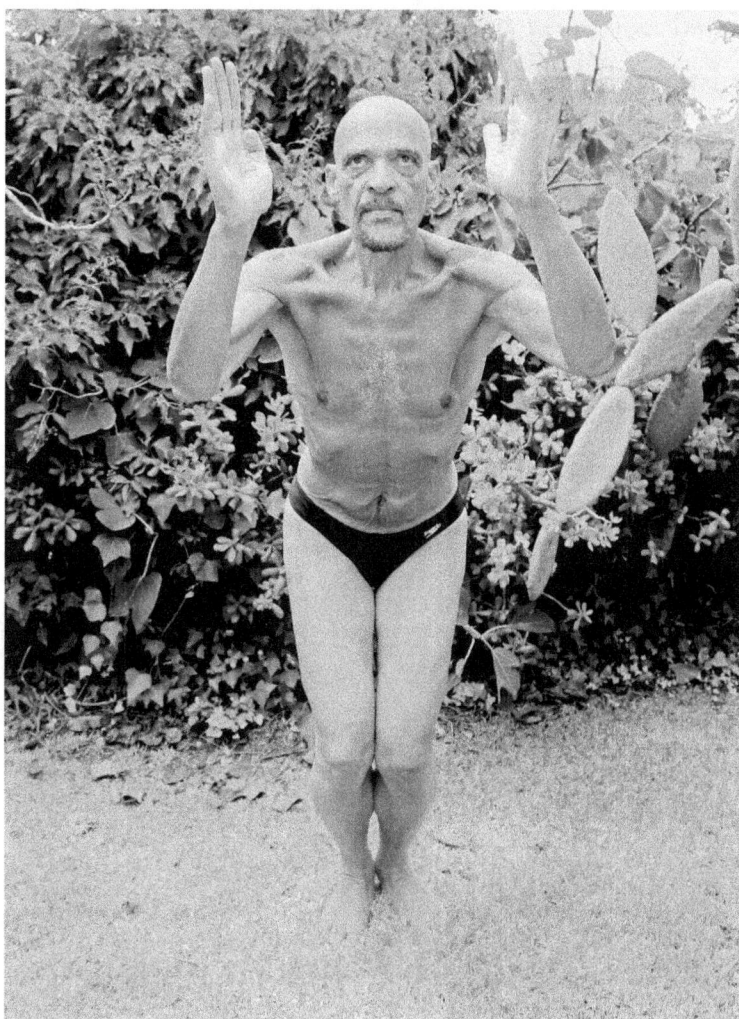

Utkat Asana (Chair Pose)

cited as one off the ways to aid in physical relief. It's just not the magic pill for it.

This semester I have chosen to place special emphasis on breathing. I have long been aware that breathing is the secret to focus, concentration, inner awareness, and attaining a true meditative state. But it's also something that must be worked at and is not automatic. I am also aware that it's not necessary to completely control the breath which is not fully possible but to experience it as a focal point to focus on awareness of self.

The most that can be safely said about yoga is that it is a mind-body practice. As such, it is regarded as both a supplement and a complement to standard treatment therapies, medication, surgery, and counseling. If practiced on a regular basis with attention paid to relaxing the mind and body through breathing, sitting quietly, and light stretching, a yoga session, can work small wonders in helping to relax and manage stress and anxiety.

* * * * *

This brings me almost full circle back to my introduction to yoga many years ago. That was the book *Raja yoga*. After I enrolled in my second yoga class, I picked up a copy again. This time I was determined to understand and hopefully incorporate into my yoga sessions the poses and movements. I say movement, because I was extremely conscious about not doing a stretch or a pose that would strain or worse pull a muscle. I am not age 29 or even 39 or even 49. I took great care to move at a slow, gentle, and as relaxed as possible pace with a pose. I had heard the agonizing stories of people who tried to do too much too soon, or watched too closely what another participant was doing, almost always someone younger, and subtly, or not so subtly, try to match or exceed their movements. This was a fatal error. It totally defeated the purpose of yoga, which, if anything, is the ultimate individual experience.

The standard make-up of my yoga classes varied little over the years. The start is the poses, or the postures, which are the movements that are what

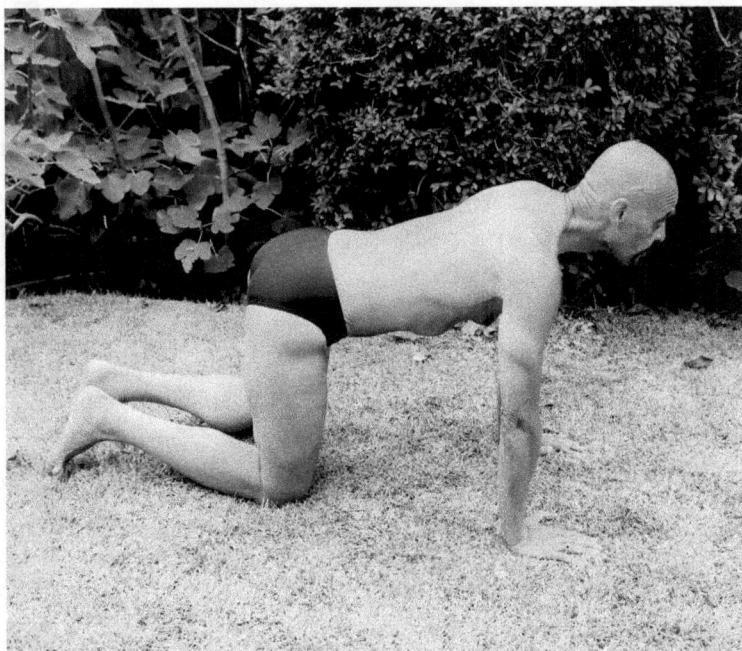

Bitil Asana (Cow Pose)

most people know and think of when they think of yoga.

The Poses. They are the series of movements that are designed to increase strength and flexibility. They can be done lying on the floor, sitting in a chair, standing up, or like a ballet dancer warming up at a railing.

The Breathing. This is the very heart and soul of yoga. Yoga instructors constantly admonish their students "don't forget to breath." This is the mantra repeated through an entire yoga session. Why? Because it helps settle and clear the mind of the emotional clutter, engenders inner tranquility, and equally important is the key to focusing your thoughts.

The Meditative. In almost all yoga sessions, time is set aside for laying or sitting quietly and focusing your thoughts or non-thoughts to quiet the mind. The trick with meditation is to try to create a moment or moments to visualize a pleasant, relaxing thought, or experience. The ideal meditation is to create an empty place or void for a moment to completely purge the problems and worries and anxieties of the day. This is a tough one for even those who are seasoned yoga participants and extremely practiced at meditation. Yet, that's the idea and the perfect tie in to yoga.

The checklist of benefits is again stress reduction, improved fitness, better physical balance, flexibility, range of motion, and strength.

*   *   *   *   *

The more controversial issue, and the one that is subject to much debate, is the role of yoga in the management of chronic physical maladies. The ones most often cited are heart disease and high blood pressure, depression, pain, anxiety, and insomnia. The debate is never-ending because there is simply no way to prove that yoga has been a proven cure for any of the major illnesses.

It's also important to remember that despite all the talk about relaxation and spiritual and mental well-being associated with yoga, it is still a physical exercise. For some it's a very intense and challenging physical workout. I have seen many participants collapse on the mat in my classes from the strain and intensity of trying to do a movement that's too hard or do it too fast, or that their body is simply not capable of doing given their level of fitness. I saw one young woman scream out and sob uncontrollably when she was unable to do one of the poses. Trying to push too hard or feeling that one must do a pose, no matter what, is a prescription for disaster.

That disaster could easily happen if someone who jumps off into yoga for the first time has any of these conditions or situations:

- A herniated disk
- A risk of blood clots
- Eye conditions, including glaucoma
- Pregnancy—although yoga is generally safe for pregnant women, certain poses should be avoided
- Severe balance problems
- Severe osteoporosis
- Uncontrolled blood pressure

There are several specific things I am working hard in an effort to master breathing as the entry point for meditative focus. One is to attain a consistent rhythm and harmony in my breath-

ing. The next is to draw mental energy and focus from the breathing. Another is to use the rhythm of my breathing to empty the mind of thoughts (clutter if you will) in order to attain mental openness and clarity. The final thing is to keep my focus on the inhaling and exhaling breaths. I am told that both are the two poles or forms of energy within our physical and subtle bodies and are the forces of positive and negative energy, the yin and yang, of our being.

*   *   *   *   *

It's imperative, of course, to avoid the more taxing poses or stretches. If there is pain at any point, it's a warning sign to ease off the accelerator or stop completely. There's absolutely no benefit from limping out of a yoga session with a pulled muscle, a cramp, or hyperventilating.

I've been fortunate to have four top notch yoga instructors. That's not always true with everyone. There are instructors and instructors. To find the right one, you got to do your homework. Ask around to find out what are the instructor's qualifications? Where did he or she train, and how long has he or she been teaching?

Does the instructor have experience working with students that have special needs or health concerns? Do they take time to ensure that the participants understand that they are not in competition with others and continually remind them to move at their own pace?

Everybody, that's every physical body, is different with different abilities and limits. This invariably requires that yoga not be seen as a one size fits all practice. Rather, yoga is something that is flexible, pliable and can be tailored to an individual's needs and abilities. I have never hesitated to ask my instructor whether a particular pose which I know was beyond my ability, could be modified. In every case, my instructors have said yes, and then demonstrated how to modify the pose to get the maximum benefit from it without risking a pull, strain or injury.

There are poses I can't do and won't try. I learned early that it is OK. You don't have to do every pose. Yoga is not a contest. It is not gymnastics event. There is no style or score points here. It's about working within your mental and physical limits and abilities, and finding the comfort level that can produce the much-vaunted relaxation, calm, and mental well-being that is the promise of yoga. The purpose is to come out of a yoga session, relaxed, not stressed. It's certainly worked for me.

3

Fact and Fiction about Yoga

I firmly believed for a long time that yoga was just another one of those fad imports from India that had folks chanting oms, gazing off into space with a blank look, and doing a bunch of pretzel like contorted twists and turns. I just knew that there couldn't be more than a relative handful of mostly health faddists, and mostly women at that, throughout the country who were into yoga. That is fiction number one about yoga.

I say number one, because like any other practice, yoga comes complete with several, if not many, fictions. I'll zero in on the most common ones. The first is its origin. Yoga originated in India, and from the little

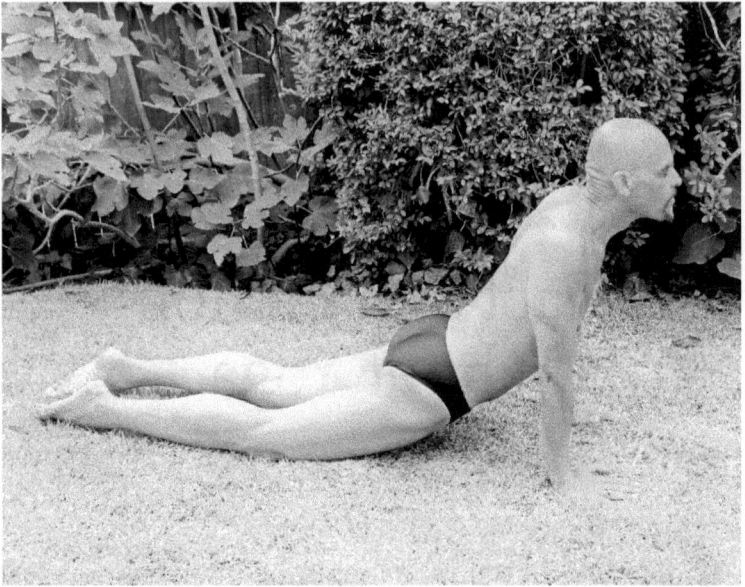

Urdhva Mukha Svan Asana (Up Dog Pose)

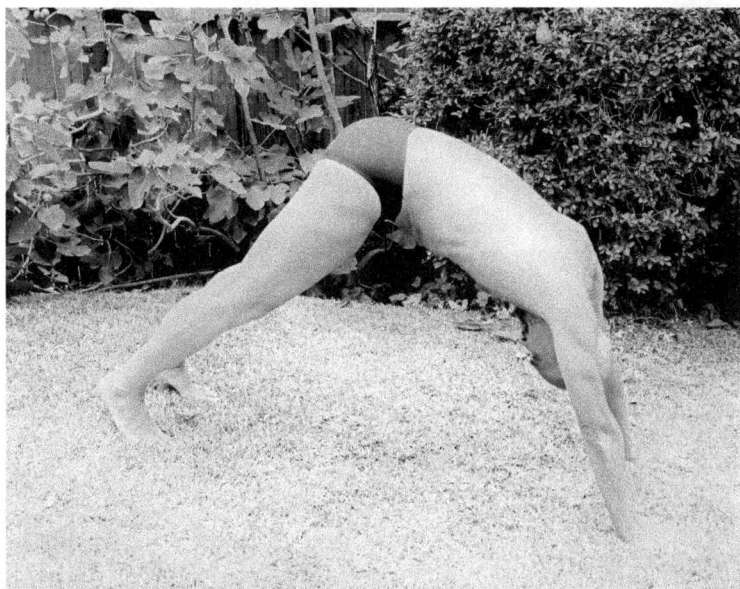

Adho Mukha Svan Asana (Down Dog Pose)

I had read initially about it, there was constant citing of Hindu or Sanskrit admonitions and verses. So, it had to be a kind of religion. In fact, this was the source of one of the controversies that periodically makes the rounds when a right-wing, evangelical preacher rails against yoga as the anti-Christ, blasphemer of Christianity. Unfortunately, some yoga devotees feed into this ignorance by continually waving the Hindu origin of yoga as if it is antithetical to Western religious beliefs and practices.

While yoga owes a profound debt to Hinduism. It has no monopoly on the evolution of yoga. There were other players in the game. They included Buddhists, Taoists, Jains, and other religious groupings. Chants, citing verses, meditation, and physical movement are also an intimate part of their beliefs and practice. When the average person thinks of yoga, they think of those twists, bends, and stretches, that are the poses. Those poses are not exclusively Indian in origin. There have been numerous add-ons, tweaks, improvisations, and modifications to yoga over the decades. They have come from modern medicine, sports, and exercise programs. Since the British held sway over India for three centuries, the Brits had some say in yoga too. That comes in the form of British calisthenics.

When yoga took off in the U.S. there were even more tweaks to it. They have their own identifiable, branded names such as yin yoga, power yoga, hot yoga, moksha/modo, bowspring, kripalu, and restorative yoga to name a few. Yoga practitioners have gotten real creative in taking the standard stuff in yoga, breathing, meditation, and the array of poses, and changing the counts in breathing, varying the sequences and postures, and how and in what position the postures should be done in.

The goal then this semester is to be continually aware of the importance of breathing in all of the yoga movements. That means incorporating breathing techniques in all of the yoga movements. It means using breathing as a focus and guide for opening my mind to positive, liberating thoughts and affirmations. Most importantly, it means using the body's most natural and life giving and affirming mechanism, and this is

breathing, to attain a true state of wellness and well-being.

* * * * *

There's still the question of whether yoga is at root a religious practice. After all, one can't totally dismiss its deep root in spiritualism. In the U.S., most yoga instructors, especially when its taught at a college, avoid like the plague, any mention of religion or spiritualism with yoga. This would open up a troubling can of worms. They would leave themselves wide open to the charge of trying to impose a new faith on students who just simply want to do yoga to lose weight, stay fit, relax, or relieve stress. Yoga instructors carefully confine their words to their students about yoga's physical and calming benefits, a way to burn some calories, and beat back stress. That's the safe approach.

Still, the common thread in the traditional forms of yoga such as *siddha yoga,* is a very explicit, and unabashed, tout of the spiritual purpose of yoga. It boldly notes the "strength and delight that come from the certainty of the divine presence within you." Then there's holy yoga which is even more explicit about God and spiritualism. It boasts that its goal is to promote "experiential worship ... to deepen people's connection to Christ." Some yoga practitiooners don't shy away from talking about spiritualism and religion in the same breath as they run their students through the poses. Even when there is not an utterance about spiritualism in a yoga session, the constant reference to relaxing the mind, listening to your breath, and closing your eyes while in a pose, suggests that one is doing a pose for more than just physical fitness or to tone a muscle. One of the major figures in the U.S. renaissance of yoga is B.K.S. Iyengar. In his "Yoga Sutras of Patanjali," he promises that yoga will bring enlightenment. Another major influential figure, K. Pattabhi Jois, in modern day yoga, tied the traditional sun salutation positions of yoga directly into Hindu texts, the *Vedas*.

* * * * *

The biggest fiction is that yoga is the magic pill to wipe away all one's cares and worries. In line with that, that one can get a pleasing, sculpted body, or failing that get back in shape by being a devotee. I'll take the stress relief part first. It's a sure bet that if you are worried about bills, a sour relationship, an illness or pain, all the breathing, up dogs and down dogs, and chair poses in one session, won't make those worries evaporate.

The real benefit of yoga is that with a little practice, concentration on the breathing and the poses, one can find momentary peace and calm. I emphasize "momentary," because like taking a pain pill, it doesn't last. You'll have to keep taking the pill to get relief. Yoga is no different. If one can come out of a session with an immediate sense of relief then yoga has more than done its job.

The same rule applies in thinking that yoga will turn one into one of those sleek muscle toned guys seem in product ads doing those yoga poses, or more likely those slender, athletic looking young women constantly depicted in articles and yoga journals and magazines. It doesn't work that way. It's going to take time, patience, and most importantly, hard work to get even close to whatever fitness level one is trying to attain.

Again, I can't tell you how many times in yoga classes, I have watched severely overweight students collapse after doing some of the most elementary of yoga poses, namely a stretch or a bend. I know that the student though well-intentioned in wanting to get into some reasonably facsimile of shape, likely won't last through the entire usually 3-month course. They are a prime candidate to drop out. The better way is to set a realistic goal for attaining a step up on the fitness scale, take it slow and easy, and really enjoy doing the movements, no matter how minimal one's effort may be.

That's not to say that even the most unfit of yoga beginners may not see a modest change after a few sessions. It's just not the norm. The fitness result will only come after months of regular practice and sticking to it. Yoga is not the instant fix that in this era of instant gratification many Americans expect and crave for.

My principal yoga instructor started the first class at the start of the semester with a yoga fitness test. As a warm-up, she walked the students through balancing poses, sit-up reps, wall stands, stretch extensions, and breath holding. The students took a precise measure of the inches and seconds they could stretch and hold their breath. In the last class at the end of the semes-

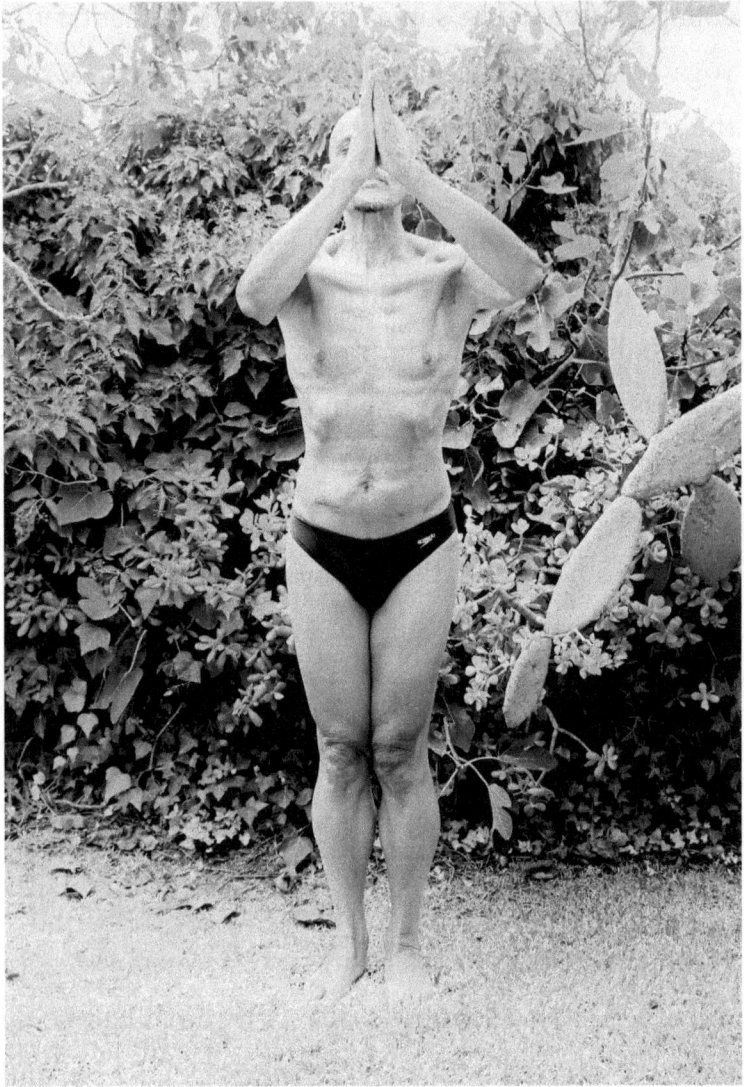

Surya Namaskar (Sun Salutation)

ter, we did the same tests. In almost every case, the changes were noticeable. We improved in all areas of fitness and flexibility. It didn't happen in weeks. It took full three months to attain these results.

The interesting thing is that in surveys of those who take yoga, the vast majority do say that they're in it to get fit, or in my case, to gain greater flexibility and muscular tone.

However, the yoga historians and scholars note that the fitness appeal of yoga was never part of the promise and vision of yoga. It was a spiritual practice in the beginning with the add on of meditation and a teaching of its philosophy, all designed to attain the heightened spiritual state of being. That was then, and there. This is the U.S. So, it's no surprise, or a heresy, that one shouldn't sweat through a yoga session and not expect to get a fitness reward from it. The yogi masters, I'm sure, wouldn't kick someone out of one of their sessions if that is what motivates them to be there.

* * * * *

The other side to the yoga boom in the U.S. is it

is now a multi-billion-dollar business. Lots of fortunes are made from yoga magazines, journals, seminars, workshops, spas, retreats, and ashrams that have sprouted up throughout the country. For a substantial price, they promise spiritual and physical rejuvenation through yoga. Then there are the smart clothing and accessories that seem almost obligatory to wear and use if you're going to look good practicing yoga. A study broke down some of the costs. It found that a studio class can cost more than $18, and a Lululemon outfit pushes $200. The requisite yoga mat which is the yoga staple can price out up to more than $100 for a top-of-the-line mat.

But let's go further into the multi-billion-dollar industry that yoga has become.

Lululemon Athletica boats that it is the "yoga-inspired athletic apparel company." It has made a mint in the past decade from its yoga geared apparel. It early on saw the boom in clothing coming and in 2006 brought on board a top executive from Rebook to oversee the apparel boom. It didn't take long for other big companies to sniff the cash that could be made from yoga and gear some of their marketing to attract some of the yoga crowd.

Ford Motor is cited as one example. It featured a woman in her 20s taking a yoga class in which she is straining to lift her body vertically into an arm-stand pose that other students around her are holding perfectly. Jewelry companies also got into the act by producing an array of necklaces and bracelets and other jewelry items with Vedic sutras and other Sanskrit sayings in and on them.

Said one manufacturer, "Each necklace comes with a message or "intention"—confidence, tranquility, happiness, performance, and so on." The companies got some of the biggest names in the motivational field such as Anthony Robbins and Deepak Chopra to hype their products. Yoga, it can truly be said, has met good old-fashioned capitalism. Whether it's a happy meeting only time will tell.

Book: Chinmoy, Sri, Yoga and the Spiritual life: The Journey of India's Soul (Aum Pubns; First edition (March 1, 1974)

Kapalbhati Pranayam: The Shining Forehead Breath

This is a simple, but effective method of doing two things to develop focus and concentration in breathing. It forces one to slow down the pace and repetition of breathing. This in turn forces the mind to focus exclusively on the inhalation and exhalation of breathing. The added beauty of this simple but effective breathing technique is that it strengthens the diaphragm and stomach muscles. The benefits then are both mental and physical.

* * * * *

One can easily get the impression from the crass commercialism in yoga product sales that yoga is more than just about fitness and spiritual growth but about dollars and cents. In other words, to get into it, as with any bought and sold commodity, it seems to many that it's going to cost some bucks. Yoga then is not for the poor but for the well-to-do and even famous.

This is another fiction. Yoga can be practiced on the grass, on a wooden floor, a rug, a carpet, in a folding chair, or just simply standing or sitting anywhere. There's no requirement that one practice yoga in a confined space, such as a studio, at inflated studio prices and membership costs. Yoga is the epitome of the individual practice. One can meditate and do the salutations and poses on the beach, in the park, in the backyard, in the home or the office.

Even more encouraging, is the spread of yoga into the prisons and low-income neighborhoods. I love to see the photos of black and Hispanic students at inner city schools in those meditative positions and going through the traditional yoga poses. I love to read about the teachers at those schools who praise the benefits of yoga for the students in engendering quiet, calm, focus, and discipline in the students.

When I see the shots of these big tough looking guys in prisons doing an up or down dog, I say to myself, "Wow, who would have ever thunk it?" This explodes the fiction that yoga is a health and wellness practice for the health conscious rich. Millions in India and other South Asian countries practiced yoga for millennia. They were anything but rich, but were among the poorest of the poor masses. There wasn't much thought, let alone talk, about yoga being solely for those who can pay.

There are many other fictions about yoga. And there will always be those who will spout them. I know, because I was one of them.

4

America's
Rush to the Mat

I long since stopped thinking of yoga as a practice for the rich, elite, mystics, and health nuts. Yoga is now wildly popular in the U.S. The figures more than bear out the spectacular emergence of yoga as a legitimate, almost made in America product. One in ten American adults have participated in a yoga activity each year since 2012.

It's not just adults. Nearly five percent of children also engaged in a yoga activity. This, according to a survey from the National Institutes of Health (NIH) and the Centers for Disease and Prevention. Other surveys put the total number of adults who have practiced yoga at one time or another, at nearly 25 million.

It's had almost as big an impact on college campuses. A decade ago one would have been hard pressed to find yoga in any college catalogue, let alone part of the PE curriculum. No more, nearly every major and small college, public and private, offers yoga classes. By the close of 2015, fitness professionals, had declared yoga the uncrowned new king on the block among sports and fitness activities in its popularity.

I can testify to the college spurt in and acceptance of yoga. When I took my second college yoga class in 2012, it was the only yoga class in the PE section in the catalogue classes. There were only a handful of students in the class. Four years later, students were practically hanging from the rafters trying to get into the class. There was an array of yoga classes in the college's course catalogue. The instructor had to turn numbers of students away. In each class, I lay elbow to elbow with students. I constantly tangled my legs with others as we worked through the various poses. This was hardly the exception. The rush to yoga was so great that a 2015 Wall Street Journal article claimed that yoga classes were so jam packed that participants were getting into shouting matches, and even physical altercations over turf.

The yoga tools of the trade—mats, blocks, straps, rollers, the fancy, spandex tights and shorts—are among the hottest selling sports items and attire. It was only a matter of time before some enterprising marketer found a hot new market for what was quickly branded "yoga pants." Then there is Yoga Journal, the yoga industry's Bible, which is published in Russia, Spain, Italy, Thailand, Brazil, and several other countries. It spotlights every nook and cranny of the yoga buying and selling craze. By 2012, it had over 2 million print readers and millions more online readers.

Each month, there has been a flock of new books and DVDs to further saturate the market. There are books for seniors, for men, the sick, the infirm, and for children. The latter is especially interesting. One author of a yoga book for children was in ecstasy in telling an interviewer that she was selling books by the truckload in the three years since her book was first published in 2009. One group of yoga converts who caught the business world's eye was Wall Street bankers and traders. They are considered among the most stressed individuals on the planet. When yoga hit big, the suit and tie crowd could be found sweating away doing their up and down dogs, twists and stretches at chic studios all around Wall Street. Business Insider reported that the gigantic Wall Street firm, Goldman Sachs, often under fire for multiple ethical and illegal trading shenanigans, even offered its employees 18 on-site yoga classes at its varied locations

I am focused on getting a handle on three areas. One is breathing. Another is meditation. The third is muscular flexibility. I have certainly gained valued information, insight, and the practical application of techniques to enhance proper breathing and to attain a better balanced meditative state. Now for flexibility.

* * * * *

The prime reason for the yoga explosion was that more and more Americans were being told that they had to lose weight, tone up those muscles, and do something, anything, to stay in shape. Yoga seemed made to order to accomplish all those things. This is only part of the reason for the surge. A lot of people,

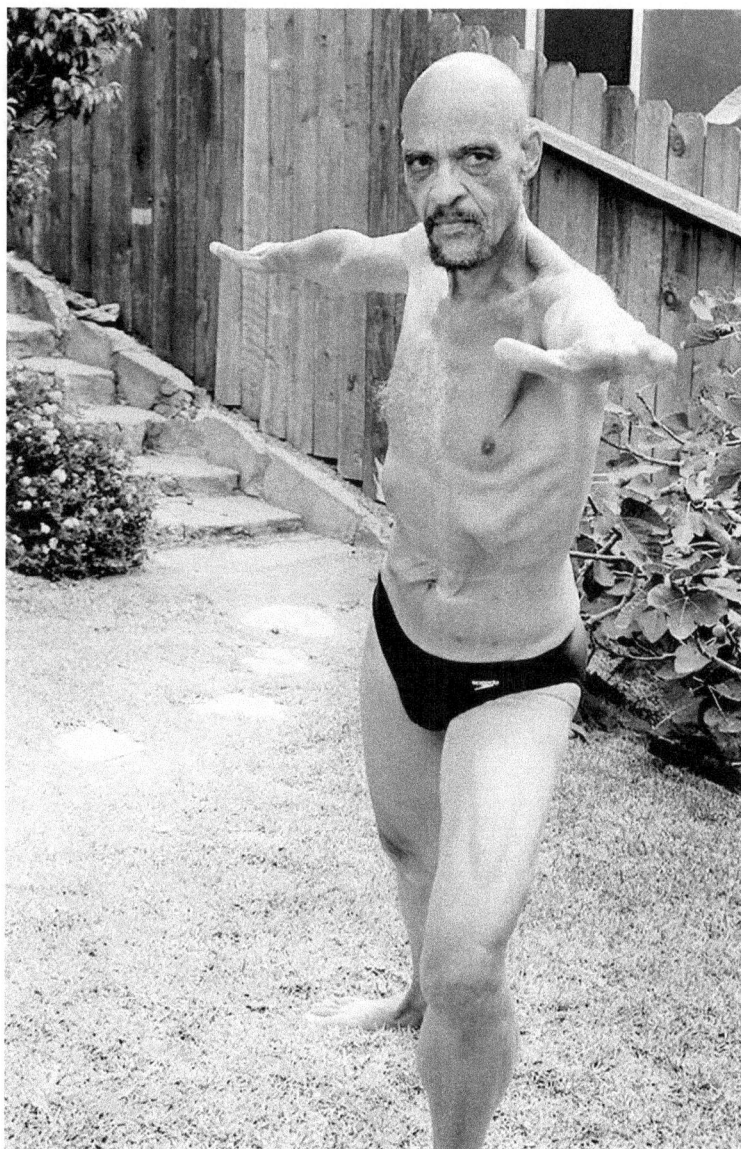

Virabhadr Asana II (Warrior II Pose)
Front

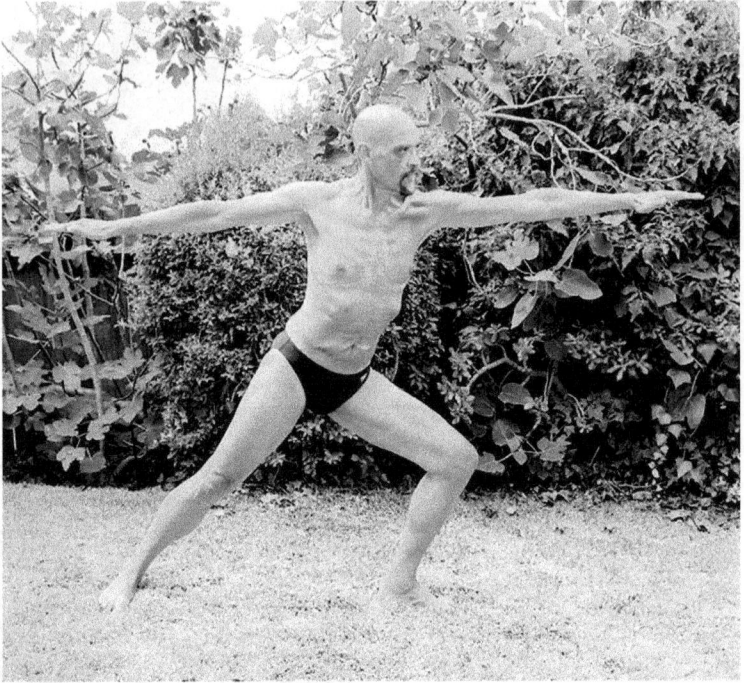

Virabhadr Asana II (Warrior II Pose)
Side

try millions, are perpetually stressed out from life's worries. Many suffer constant bouts of anxiety, and are being warned by an increasing number of medical professionals, that stress can trigger serious physical illness and ailments. Some doctors are even more blunt. They label stress as a potential killer. There are even studies that seem to bear out the suspected connection between stress and physical health.

The answer for millions is to cram their medicine chests with a pharmacy worth of stress and anxiety relief medications. The problem with that is that medication has a nasty little byproduct. It's called addiction. That's not all. The more medication one takes the less effective it can be. That requires popping more pills and more potent doses of them to get relief.

There is a break point to this. A lot of doctors who previously laughed away the notion that a pill can do anything for anxiety, now started preaching the benefits of exercise and physical activity as the key to knocking down the stress levels. It was only a short step from this to discovering yoga as potentially a great natural therapy tool to keep the body and mind on the right track. Yoga got a further boost when the federal government stepped in 2012, and agreed to expand coverage to pay for those with heart ailments and who are taking yoga as part of their cardiac rehabilitation regimen.

Some doctors are now enthusiastic cheerleaders for alternative medicine, "I've always thought that it's not a matter of if we are going to include yoga and mindfulness techniques in health care, it's always been when, and the when has arrived," says M. Mala Cunningham, a psychologist at the University of Virginia who founded a program to certify yoga instructors and medical professionals to use such techniques with cardiac patients. She was right and with that yoga in effect now carried the official imprimatur of the government.

The second semester the focus was on the meditative aspects of yoga. My focus was on concentration, relaxation, and freeing the mind, body and spirit to prepare myself for a meditative experience that would truly free the mind of the mental baggage and clutter. The continuous positive affirmations from the instructor was

**and has been tantamount to a guided medita-
tion session each class. It has been immensely
instructive and guiding.**

*   *   *   *   *

Despite the doctor's prescient take on the coming
of yoga as an accepted wellness aid. The skeptics still
abound. Most doctors, and standard medical practitioners, still regard it as only a "complementary" health
practice. The National Institute of Health uses that
term in its periodic reports on the efficacy of alternative medicine. The NIH's Center for Complementary
and Integrative Health said this about yoga, "it might
improve quality of life; reduce stress; lower heart rate
and blood pressure; help relieve anxiety, depression,
and insomnia; and improve overall physical fitness,
strength, and flexibility." It is no accident that the first
word out of the center's descriptive box about yoga is
"might." It notes that studies of yoga for asthma sug-
gest no benefit; and that studies in arthritis patients
have had mixed results.

The occasional toss of cold water on yoga has done
nothing to dampen its popularity and conversely the

money train it rides on. It can be said that yoga has come out of the closet of the fringe few. It is now an accepted, and very lucrative, exercise and business. As long as stress and anxiety hammer millions of Americans and they are desperate to do something about it, as well as their physical unfitness, yoga has nowhere to go but up, up, and up in popularity. This insures that many more will sing the praises of yoga as the new elixir to solve their ailments and woes.

5

Only the Mat Was Black

I went through a litany of stereotypes, conceptions, misconceptions, ill-informed notions, and just plain ignorance in my thinking about yoga in the years before my awakening. By far, the two biggest misconceptions I had were on, that it is a woman's thing. In the magazine and newspaper articles and promotional stuff I saw on yoga, it was always young, chic, slender young women, going through the poses. The other major misconception I had was that they weren't just young sculpted women. They were white women.

From this, I concluded that yoga was a practice where African-Americans, Hispanics, and other mi-

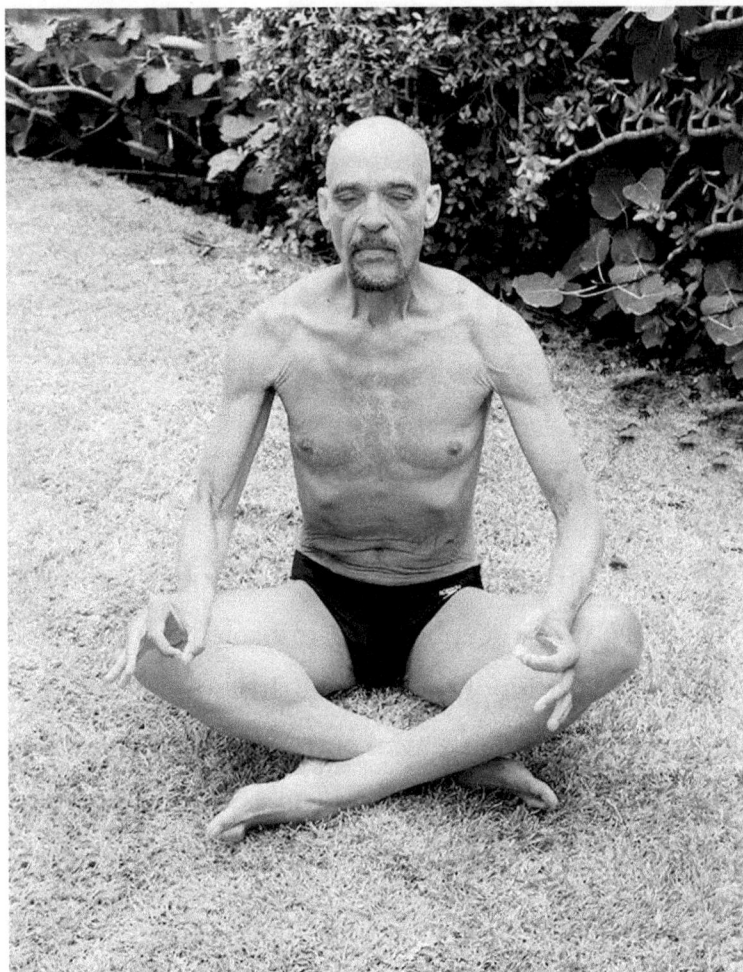

Sukh Asana (Meditation Pose)

norities, would not only not be found in studios doing down dogs. Worse, in a subtle and no so subtle
way, they were not really wanted in those studios. A
few years later, I read an article entitled, "Is American
Yoga Racist?" The author told of a yoga studio in Santa
Barbara, California, where the owners got the bright
idea of trying to attract more blacks to join the studio. They put up a big poster inviting the black locals
to visit the studio for a free session. The session was
billed as "Ghetto-Fabulous."

They did not do it as a prank, or out of malice, or
just to be cute. They really didn't see anything offen-
sive in this since the ancient stereotype in America is
that all blacks live in run down inner-city neighborhoods, attend grossly failing public schools, and are
eternal purveyors of crime, drugs and gang violence.
However, what was unpardonable is that the women
drove the promotion by flipping imagined gang signs,
and asking anyone who took up the offer of the "ghet-
to fabulous" free session to wear their hair and dress
in attire that they imagined is the regalia of African-
Americans.

Any other time and place, such a crass, and grotesque mockery of blacks, would have ignited a fire-storm of rage. Almost certainly the offenders would backpedal fast and sweat through a litany of *mea culpas*. However, there was not a peep of outrage or protest within the yoga world about it. The question that was never clearly answered then or now, was this simply the foolish, stupid, act, of a handful of ill-informed women that flew under the radar scope of yoga aficionados? Or, did they regard this as an aberration by a group of women, at one studio, at one place, and at one time, and not worth the bother of taking them to task?

It certainly was a golden opportunity to bare the chest about ways to make the practice more inclusive to African-Americans and other minorities. It was also an opportunity to dispel the prevailing notion that yoga is a closed-door shop to all other than well-to-do whites.

This semester I have chosen to place special emphasis on breathing. I have long been aware that breathing is the secret to focus, concentra-tion, inner awareness, and attaining a true medi-

tative state. It's also something that has to be worked at and is not automatic. I am also aware that it's not necessary to completely control the breath which is not fully possible but to experience it as a focal point to focus on. There are several specific things I am working hard in an effort to master breathing as the entry point for meditative focus. One is to attain a consistent rhythm and harmony in my breathing.

* * * * *

There is no study or survey that breaks down by race and ethnicity the number of African-Americans among the nearly 25 million Americans who practice yoga. We are left with trying to guestimate the number. Since for the most part the pictures and promotional ads and spots that one sees of yoga practitioners and participants are of mostly young, chic dressed, white women, it's easy to conclude that the numbers overall of Blacks and Hispanics, in particular, in yoga are still small. It's true, there has been a concerted effort by some African-American yoga teachers to take yoga into inner city neighbors, and have introduced the practice to kids in a few schools in these neighborhoods. There are also a few yoga classes that are held in a handful of prisons. They are the rare exceptions, so rare, that they invariably make news, because they are such an anomaly.

There are two prime reasons why yoga has not gripped the imagination of more African-Americans, Hispanics and minorities. The first is simple economics and accessibility. A yoga studio in an African-American or Hispanic neighborhood is a rarity. The colleges that offer yoga courses are largely removed from these communities.

It costs nothing for someone to sit on the sand, the grass, or the floor in their apartment dressed in whatever they have on at the time to work through some yoga poses and to meditate. However, the ubiquitous promotion and marketing of yoga attire, sessions, accessories and studios, deliberately convey the message that yoga is indeed costly. After all, it's about selling a product. If one is in the business of clothing design or manufacturing and part of their product line is athletic wear, you're going to put a top dollar price tag on that garment. With the popularity of yoga, comes high demand for the right attire to look right while going through a session. It's not going to be cheap.

Then there's the yoga studios. Again, they are few and far between in predominantly Black and Hispanic neighborhoods. Yet, they are all over the joint in predominantly white suburban neighborhoods and near major university campuses. A session at any one of them can be pricey. At the suburban yoga studio where I attend classes from time to time, more often than not, I find myself negotiating with the owner to get the cost down. In return, I offer to do some promotions for the studio on my weekly public affairs radio show. It's a trade-off they agree to, but that's for me, because I have something to offer in return. This something is a radio spot and free radio promotion. That can translate out into more customers and more membership sales for their studio.

* * * * *

The second major problem is the cultural disconnect that has become a self-fulfilling prophecy. It goes like this. Very few Blacks are interested in yoga. Very few Blacks are in classes, or at yoga studios. Ergo, very few Blacks are interested in yoga or will attend any yoga classes or sessions at studios. This is akin to the argument that raged for decades that Blacks were no good at swimming or tennis or golf because they were practically non-existent in those sports. We see where that argument went when Blacks saw models of success in those sports. Now as if by magic, Blacks are seen everywhere on golf and tennis courts, and diving into swimming pools. The issue is exposure, and once the barriers come down, and Blacks and Hispanics can see models of success that look like them, it is off to the races.

Yoga is no different. If there are teachers who teach at inner city schools, and recreation centers that routinely offer yoga classes, and people can practice yoga in parks in inner-city neighborhoods, Blacks and Hispanics will be there. If it is included in PE courses in middle and high schools, more and more Black and Hispanic kids will take it up.

* * * * *

There were two challenges in using yoga techniques and postures to attain greater flex-

ibility. The first challenge was age. The inescapable fact is that with the aging process there is flexibility loss. Obviously, the average 60-year-old can't move the muscles and joints as fluidly as a 20-year-old. The second challenge was I have been a runner for many years. I have run 7 marathons and countless 5 and 10K races and I still run five days a week. Flexibility has always been a huge issue with runners—of any age. We just simply do not pay enough attention to prolonged and proper stretching before and after runs. Yoga was a partial antidote to that.

The flip side of this is that if *Yoga Journal,* and the numerous other yoga magazines and publications see that Blacks and Hispanics in sizeable numbers buy their products, then marketing companies and advertisers will shift gears offer night and feature more people of color in their ads. It's not altruism but dollars.

This is exactly what happened with just about every major corporation in America in the 1990s. They discovered that minorities were major consumers too.

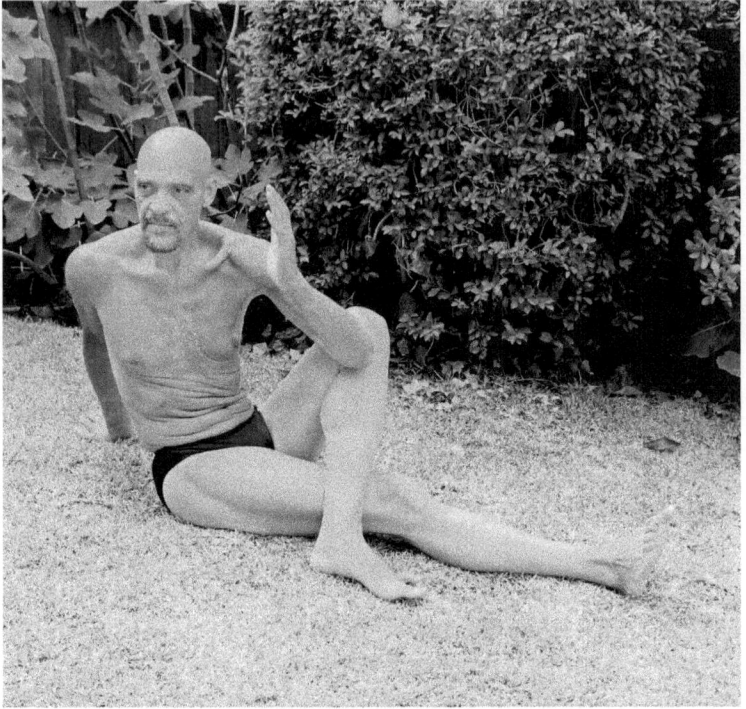

Ardha Matsyendra or Bharad Vaja Asana
(Sitting Half Spine Twist Posture)
Front

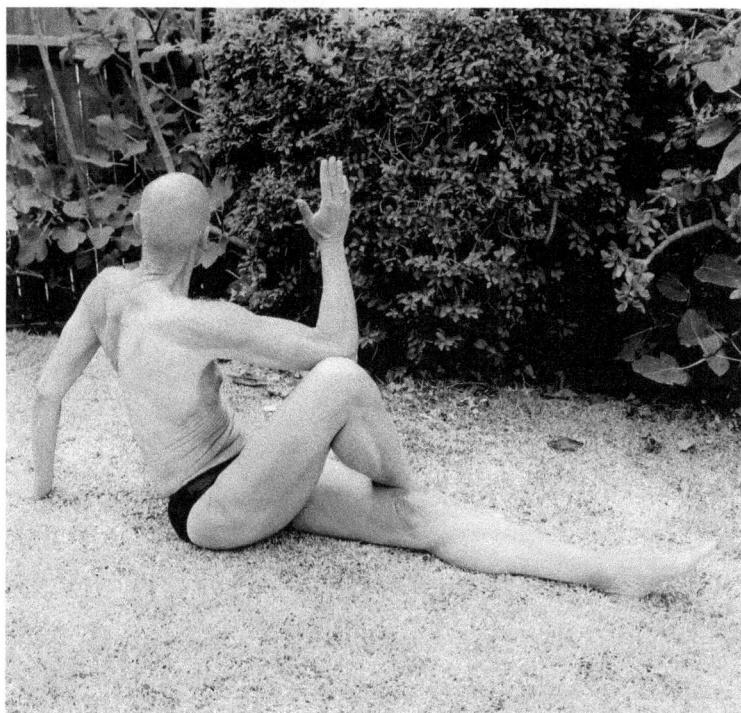

Ardha Matsyendra or Bharad Vaja Asana
(Sitting Half Spine Twist Posture)
Back

One cannot turn on the TV now without seeing droves of Blacks and Hispanics and Asians buying cars, computers, clothes, guzzling beer, and just about any other product that's on the market in commercials. The major firm's marketing epiphany came when they realized there's a big, untapped market out there among minorities who buy a lot of their products, and will buy even more of them if they are constantly beat over the head with ads that come complete with faces that look like theirs.

Big business also realized that there are a lot of Blacks and Hispanics who make a lot of money. They are not just the big name, high profile Hollywood stars, musicians, and athletes. But a lot of Black and Hispanic business persons, professionals and highly paid skilled workers. They have the income to indulge themselves and buy luxury goods. They need to unwind too, stay in physical shape, and bring some calmness to their minds too. They have the money to spend on a practice that promises to help them do just that.

There's one other problem in the quest to attain true diversity in yoga. The problem is buried deep in yoga itself. Yoga's roots are firmly planted in spiritualism. There is no color, gender, or even class distinction in principle made. The spiritualism in yoga eschews human foibles, desires, prejudices, and divisions. It is supremely individualistic. It is designed to promote spiritual depth and mental well-being. It is non-judgmental about human failures and offers as an antidote tolerance and even acceptance of the world as it is. The focus remains on instilling internal, rather than external, peace and harmony in an individual.

Unlike Western Christianity that has erected color barriers and divisions, yoga philosophy and practice is color-neutral. It is also not a practice that seeks to convert and proselyte like Islam. This entails inculcating its potential converts in the dogma of the religion. It is no accident that many of the top long-term yoga practitioners are not conversant on the hot button political and social issues of the day, let alone directly involve themselves in political actions.

One of my principal yoga instructors frankly told me that she wasn't really political, and did not listen to public affairs radio talk shows that focused on political issues. She was not atypical. She saw yoga as a refuge from the turmoil of the world. A big part of that turmoil is, of course, racial conflict.

*   *   *   *   *

There's even some speculation that since yoga is a product of Eastern religion and religious practices, it provides a convenient cover to ignore the problems of race, gender and class that are endemic in the West. This is pure conjecture. The truth is yoga is a practice grounded in the promotion of spiritual and mental well-being. There is nothing inherent in Eastern culture, religions and sects, that explicitly denigrates or excludes other cultures and religious practices.

If race is an issue within yoga, the blame lay exclusively with those who practice it. There's the old adage that Islam, Christianity, Judaism, Buddhism, and other religions are a work of beauty and marvel in principle and on paper. The problem is that Muslims, Christians, Jews, Buddhists and those of other religions muck it on in practice.

Many black writers, who either have studied yoga as an academic exercise, or actually practice it and have created their own online blog, *Black Yogi,* almost universally finger point either the yoga commercial industry, yoga publications, or the yoga instructor as the ones who have set racial boundaries, either consciously or deliberately, within the world of yoga. They have brought their own racial biases to a field which by definition has none. The spate of articles that have appeared in major publications such as *Forbes* and the *Huffington Post* that have probed the issue of racism and yoga, zeroed in on racial bias perpetuated by individuals as the culprit.

There are two things that virtually insure yoga will not be the near exclusive preserve of toney whites in the years to come. One is yoga's history. It has been pliable and adaptable enough to accommodate tweaks and modifications to it. It has served as a big tent for the many varied types of yoga and the varied ways they are taught.

The other is the changing ethnic demographics of America. By 2050 America will no longer be a majority white country, if current population trends hold up. By then yoga will have millions of new adherents to draw from. It's inevitable that a big portion of those new devotees will be Blacks and Hispanics and other minorities. When that happens, it no longer will be said that in yoga only the mat was black.

6

Where are the Guys?

I can't forget my first yoga instructor's words when I casually mentioned that I was surprised at the number of men in the class. She said, "It seems unusual because men think that yoga is for women." She quickly added that the gender identification of yoga as a "woman's thing" flies in the face of the history of yoga. For the greater part of that history yoga teachers and practitioners were men. She knew of what she spoke. She had spent a year in India studying and practicing yoga and she said that not only were her teachers, men, but often she was the only woman in the yoga classes and retreats.

Yet, the reality is that the great majority of yoga students and participants are women. The figures bear that out. The most comprehensive study conducted on the state of yoga in the U.S. by *Yoga Journal* and Yoga Alliance in 2016 found that over 70 percent of those practicing yoga are women. One doesn't need the numbers to confirm the obvious. Women are the driving force in yoga in the U.S. They spend tens of millions on the fancy attire, the mats, and other accessories. They are the ones whose pictures fill page after page of yoga magazines, journals and other publications. They are the ones who pack the yoga classes at colleges and at private studios.

My instructor's quip that most men think that yoga is for women is a double-edged sword for yoga and for men. The one side of it is that the thought of yoga as for women only is so deep seated in the thinking of many men and women that it's become a disincentive, even a barrier, for many men to take up the practice. It seems somehow unmanly to be sandwiched in between women on a yoga mat doing those contortions, and twists, bends, and stretches that are the staple of yoga. Many women are willing to go explore new frontiers and adaptable to new experiences, such as yoga. Many men, in contrast, are more guarded and

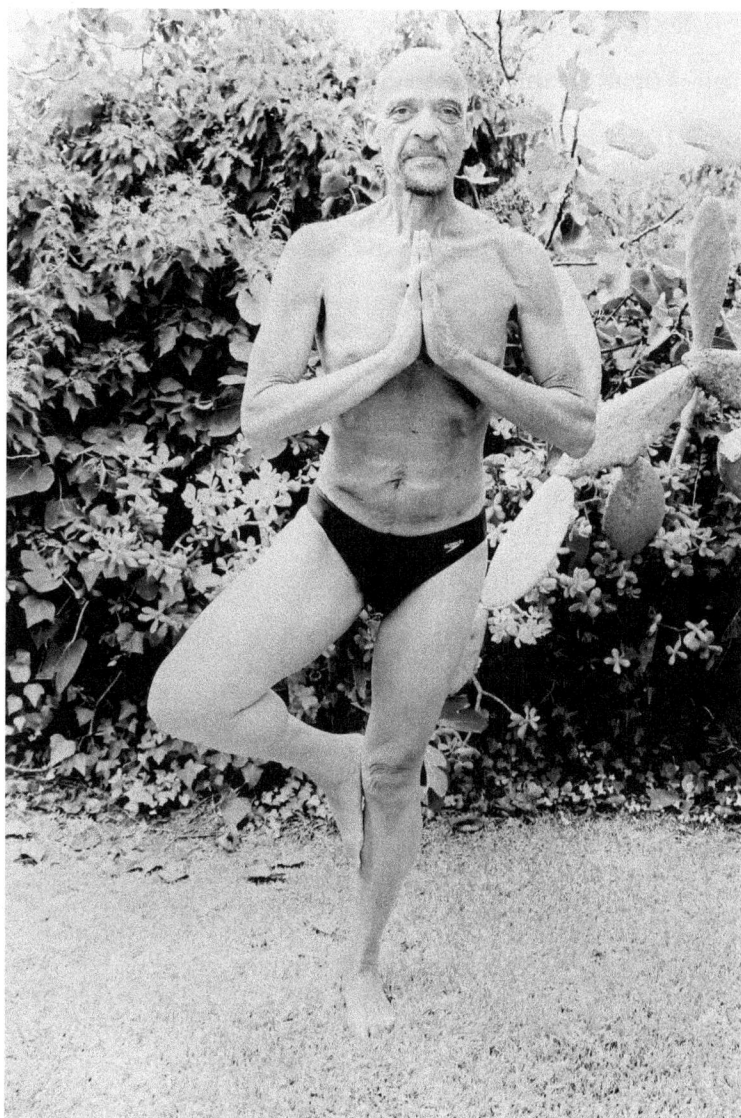

Vriksha Asana (Tree Pose)

protective of their image as aggressive and domineering. Yoga doesn't lend itself to either.

The other side to the sword is that the narrow gender typecasting of yoga has prevented many men from enjoying the benefits of yoga. The men who have taken the plunge, and the number stands at over 20 percent of the yoga participants, include football, basketball and soccer players and weight lifters. They swear that it has helped them with flexibility, muscle tone and served as a stress reliever. Many of these guys who are down dogging are hulking physical specimens. No one challenges or questions their manhood.

The dangling question then given the unquestioned benefits of yoga, is just why aren't more men in the classes and studios? The answer can be summed up in this checklist of excuses typically given:

- I am not flexible enough to do yoga
- I will look stupid
- It looks painful
- Why waste time on an activity that doesn't have a score and a winner
- Yoga isn't exercise

- Just not interested
- It's a girl thing

The goal then this semester is to be continually aware of the importance of breathing in all of the yoga movements. That means incorporating breathing techniques in all of the yoga movements. It means using breathing as a focus and guide for opening my mind to positive, liberating thoughts and affirmations. Most importantly, it means using the body's most natural and life giving and affirming mechanism and this is breathing, to attain a true state of wellness and well-being.

* * * * *

Excuse number 7 is the last in this checklist for a good reason. It's still the runaway number one reason why more guys aren't on the mats. In fairness, some men have been scared away from it because of the perceived risks of injury. They have heard the horror stories about men who have suffered painful and nagging pulls and strains doing yoga poses. There is even re-

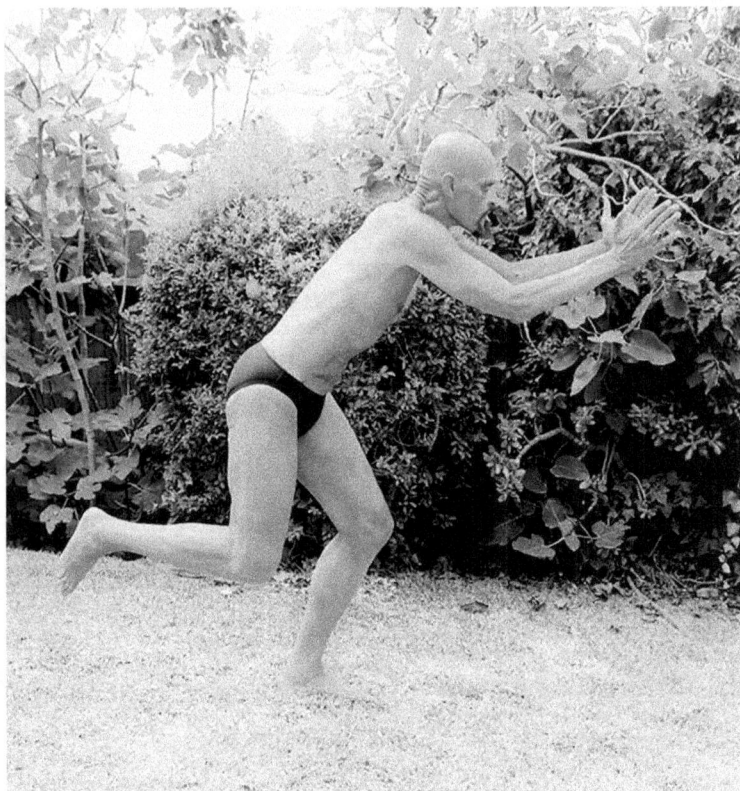

Virabhadr Asana III (Warrior III Pose)

search to back up the notion that men are more prone to yoga related injuries. This has less to do with men's supposed greater inflexibility, then in trying to do too much, too soon, and too aggressively. The injuries are due in part to impatience, in part to ego, and in part to the need to turn everything they engage in into competition. In the case of yoga, seeing it as another form of sporting competition.

I'll circle back to the more than 20 percent of yoga participants who are men. The reasons many of them are just as passionate about yoga as women aren't hard to find. Those reasons debunk the gender myths about yoga. It is every bit a full body workout. It is not just a way to tone muscles but can also build and strengthen muscles too. The continual up and down movement in the poses can also be an intense aerobic workout. Despite the claim that yoga can be a way to lose weight, I don't think that is totally true. If any weight is lost through yoga, it more likely is due to a change or modification of diet, in correspondence with the practice. If one can drop a pound or two after a few weeks with yoga then that's all the better. I'm willing to give yoga the credit.

The major complaint that yoga can lead to injury and the reason for that is that men are less flexible than women can't be shrugged off. The risk can be minimized merely by seeing yoga for what it is. That is a gentle form of body movement, and not rush things. When men bring that mindset to yoga, the risk of injury is minimized and increases the range of motion and suppleness of the muscles. In the post fitness test my instructors give in their yoga classes, I'm always amazed and gratified, that after three months of yoga in the class, I can actually touch my toes without bending my knees when I do the toe touch test. Medical experts confirmed that a wider range of motion increases access to more muscle fibers, as well as enlarges muscles. The take away from this is that yoga prevents injuries because the muscles are well-stretched and are able to recover more quickly.

I see no physical risks in this type of breathing technique. In fact, the slow, methodical repetitive nature of this breathing virtually insures that this does not cause undue physical stress during the exhalation of the diaphragm.

I inhale as normal through the nostrils. I try to take in as much air as possible—filling up the lungs so to speak—and letting the chest contract. The exhalation is also through the nostrils but with a mild even exaggerated degree of force and making sure that I use my stomach muscles to aid in the exhalation (for added force). I repeat this as many times as I feel comfortable with. That's usually 10 to 12 minutes.

* * * * *

There is one thing about yoga that if promoted more extensively could be a huge selling point to get more men into yoga. This is the promise that it will make men tigers in the bedroom. A 2010 study, offered a tantalizing hint that this could indeed be the case. It found that regular yoga exercise improved all domains of sexual function in men. The breathing techniques and concentration practiced in yoga seemed to help men better channel their sexual energy.

I want to see more studies done on this before I dash to tout yoga as a big booster of sexual prowess. If there's truth that it does, I still wouldn't promote it as a prime reason for men to hit the mat. One of the two main reasons I embraced yoga is because it increased my flexibility. The other was what yoga remains. It's an exercise that can promote calm and well-being after a stressful day. The movements combined with the breathing properly can induce a pleasant feel that restores and reenergize the old brain cells.

*   *   *   *   *

I can talk all day about the whys and the wherefores of why more men should be in yoga classes. However, there is still will be many who pose the counter intuitive argument: Why should I do yoga, when there are other ways to stay in shape, to stay fit, and reduce stress? These activities don't expose me to the potential embarrassment of being stuck in a class with mostly women. That's a tough argument to get around. In fact, some men go further in the push back. They say stop, enough with trying to turn guys into yoga devotees. Yoga is clearly something that many are uncomfortable with. Or put even more bluntly, they say, stop trying to make more men do yoga.

I won't counter this with more talk about the health benefits of yoga, since men can get those benefits in many other physical activities. Instead, how about this. If you can get or maintain a muscle toned look, and know that some of the most muscular and physically imposing men, actually do yoga as a supplement to maintain muscle tone, then is that a compelling enough reason to consider yoga? If there were photos routinely run in yoga magazines and journals and in advertisements of men, muscular men, doing yoga and looking like they enjoy it, that would make the powerful statement that yoga is not solely for women.

Many of those photos that promote yoga could be of men in the one sport that is near universally regarded as the ultimate in male muscularity and toughness. That's pro football. In 2015, there were enough NFL stars taking up yoga that it caught the eye of feature writers in mainstream publications such as the *New York Times.* The articles ticked off the names of some of the best-known players in the NFL who were either taking yoga on their own, or taking it under the private tutelage of a yoga instructor.

One instructor who travelled on the road to some of the games with the players said that she had 17 pro players from various teams that she would take through the steps. The ball players she trained praised to the skies the benefits that they felt they got from yoga. They included the standard stuff—greater flexibility, the ability to recover from injuries faster, improved focus, and greater sense of relaxation, calmness and well-being. She walked through the steps that she uses with the players starting with what's called "the wheel." This was designed by two top international yoga teachers,

She explains how the wheel works, "The traditional class starts with breathing and warm-up, But I let them roll out the wheel; they usually are coming off a hard practice, so it will relax the body, help them feel mellow and calm. Then we go into breathing; I stress breathing with the guys — it helps them on the field and to remain calm in a stressful situation., We do some flow sequences, some yoga poses."

She took particular note of the change it has made in their lives, "They walk into our sessions with the stress of it. I can see it on their faces at any session, the tiredness. But by the time they breathe and do a little bit of yoga, there is something that disappears, and a calm that comes from them. The mental wellness of yoga is by far the biggest part for an athlete. It gives a Zen calmness their sport doesn't teach them."

The more interesting aspect of the spotlight put on football guys who are into yoga is that the NFL had already beaten the feature writers to a showcase of the players doing yoga. NFL films did a special in 2013 on former Jacksonville Jaguars linebacker Keith Mitchell's almost messianic mission to spread the benefits of yoga to other pro football players and other athletes. Mitchell told how his discovery of yoga had helped in his recovery both mentally and physical after a career ending injury on the field. The NFL special on yoga put the league's official stamp of approval on it. It was now officially recognized as a practice that big, strong, tough guys could readily embrace.

* * * * *

The Zen calmness that the yoga trainer talked about in her training sessions with the football guys also strikes to another reason why men work out. It's not just because they want to look good, but they want to feel good too. It's about appearance, and while this entails how someone looks physically, appearance is how someone think others see them, and how they want the world to see them. This is huge with men. You can call it vanity, ego or society's rigid, dated, and stereotypical take on male prowess. Yet, they are still potent parameters of how many men think they should look and act.

Yoga will always be principally regarded by men who take it up as a form of physical fitness, a way to stay or get in shape. This is not a bad thing. In fact, it's one of the strong points of yoga that can be exploited for all its worth to affirm with men that it's OK to be in a yoga class no matter how many women there are in it. When men walk into a yoga class or studio, they can say to themselves I feel good about being here, then it's a good fit for me, because it's just like going to the gym, and when I come out of the class I'll feel exactly like I do when I come from the gym, with all of the perceived benefits I get from it.

The caveat is that yoga can't be pushed on men. No amount of beating men over the head with the argument that it's nonsense to think of yoga as a woman's thing will do much to convince many men that it isn't. Yoga, it can't be said enough is an individual practice, and an individual will get out of it what he or she puts into it. This should be the real selling point of yoga for men. If they can lift a barbell and gain a bit more muscle mass, then they can do a tree pose to gain a bit more muscle tone. It's just a matter of one picking their preference for what will get the job done.

It's not an insurmountable challenge to get more men into yoga. In fact, studies find, and a look in many yoga classes will confirm, that many of the growing number of Americans who practice yoga are men. They understand that yoga can do much for them. They embrace it as part of their overall fitness program. They are living breathing proof that yoga is not just a "girl's thing."

Conclusion

The State of Yoga and Me

I still marvel at the thought that five years after I walked into a yoga class at my local community college that I am still just as enthused and impassioned about yoga as I was at the first class. If anyone had asked me before entering that first class the question, "Who would you say would be among the last persons on the planet you know who would take up yoga," I would unhesitatingly answer, "me." Just about every negative that has been said about yoga, I believed.

However, the beauty is that those negatives not only were quickly dispelled, but in the years that I have practiced yoga, they have been stood on their head.

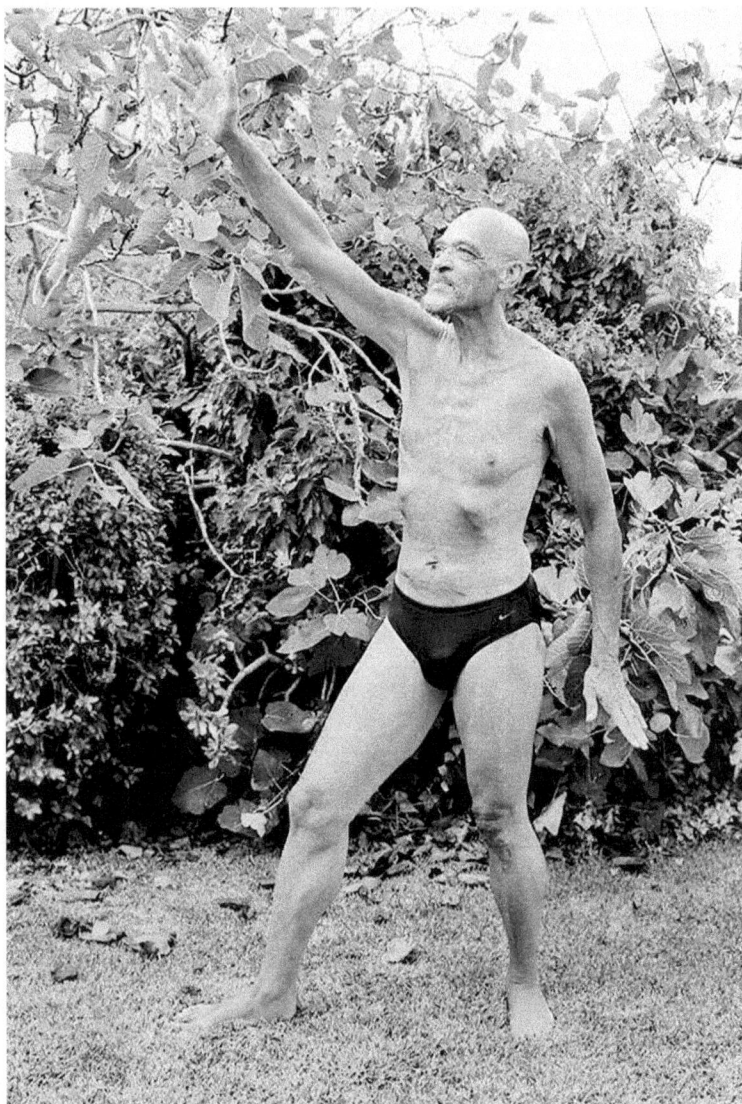

Virabhadr Asana I (Warrior I Pose)

Yoga is manly. It is not an injury maker. It does not make a seemingly inflexible man seem less flexible. It is not for young athletic white women. It is not for rich, whites only.

Yoga opened a new world, a world of infinite possibilities to attain fitness, calm, and spiritual growth. It shoved me out of my comfort zone physically and mentally. I am very careful not to go overboard and ascribe all kinds of elixir powers to yoga which it does not possess. I keep it in perspective and see it as the doctors like to say a "complement" to my other life's activities.

I like the conventional, literal meaning of this sutra. That is vritti means whirlpool. This is an appropriate definition and by extension this yoga sutra. Our minds are a continual whirlpool of ideas, thoughts, and reflections. Flowing from this mental turbulence are our doubts, worries, concerns, preoccupations and stresses. The prime goal and challenge is how to "silence" or calm or even tame this whirlpool of mental turbulence. This is the key

to engendering, or perhaps entering is a more accurate way of stating it, a heightened state of mental peace, tranquility, and harmony. According to the philosophy of this sutra, this is the direct pathway to attaining enlightenment about being, self, the world within and without.

* * * * *

I can't stop here. I figured that if I were going to be a devotee of yoga that I should know as much about it as possible. That is, its history, its philosophy, and how it has been used and even misused. So, I hit the books on it and read and studied as much as I could about it. Fortunately, with the tremendous surge in interest in yoga in the past two decades in the U.S., there is a wide body of literature on yoga to give a full and comprehensive picture of the state of yoga in the U.S. today.

This picture of the state of yoga in the U.S. is on display in the study 2016 Yoga in America Study Conducted by *Yoga Journal* and Yoga Alliance. The study revealed:

- There are 36.7M US yoga practitioners, up from 20.4M in 2012
- 34 percent of Americans say they are somewhat or very likely to practice yoga in the next 12 months – equal to more than 80 million Americans
- Students spend $16B/year on classes, gear, and equipment, up from $10B in 2012
- Women represent 72 percent of practitioners; men, 28 percent
- The top five reasons for starting yoga are: flexibility (61 percent), stress relief (56 percent), general fitness (49 percent), improve overall health (49 percent), and physical fitness (44 percent)
- 86 percent of practitioner's self-report having a strong sense of mental clarity, 73 percent report being physically strong, and 79 percent give back to their communities – all significantly higher rates than among non-practitioners

For me, the skeptic, who once ridiculed the claim of yoga to be a positive force for physical, mental, and spiritual regeneration, it has indeed been an odd, but fascinating journey through the yoga experience. It's a journey that has more than delivered on the promise of yoga to enhance my health and well-being, if given a chance. I did and I'm eternally thankful for it.

Abraham Lincoln is reputed to have once said that "a person can be about as happy as they want to be." I thought of this Lincolnesque aphorism when reading about this sutra. Now Lincoln as far as we know never studied or practiced yoga. But he discovered the eternal truth of this sutra and that is one can attain true contentment by thinking, focusing on and embodying in one's being in a happy or joyful mental state. Turning doom and gloom on its head and find joy both within and without whether it's a walk in the park on a cool, breezy, but sunny day or simply looking for and discovering joy in our day-to-day relationships and life. Another way to put it is this perception becomes reality. If we think joy and contentment constantly we will find it and attain it.

Finally, it means acceptance of those things that can't be changed, and changing those

things that can. First and foremost, that means our thoughts, perceptions, and being.

Namaste

The Asanas

Sanskirt Name (English Translation)

Surya Namaskar (Sun Salutation)

Adho Mukha Svan Asana (Down Dog Pose)

Akarna Dhanur Asana (Shooting Bow Posture)

Ardha Chandra Asana (Half Moon Posture)

Ardha Hal Asana (Half Plow Pose)

Ardha Matsyendra or

Bharad Vaja Asana (Sitting Half Spine Twist Posture)

Baddha Kona Asana (Restrained Angle Posture)

Bala Asana (Child Posture)

Bhujang or Nag Asana (Cobra or Snake Pose)

Bitil Asana (Cow Pose)

Chakra Asana (Wheel Posture)

Dhanur Asana (Bow Posture)

Ekapada Asana (One-legged Posture)

Garuda Asana (Half Spinal Twist Posture)

Gomukha Asana (Cow Face Posture)

Hala Asana (Plow Posture)

Hasta Pada Angusta Asana (Fish Posture)

Katichalana Asana (Cross-leg Twisting Pose)

Mandnuk Asana (Frog Pose)

Marjaria Asana (Cat Pose)

Nataraja Asana (King of the Dance Posture)

Nauv Asana (Boat Pose)

Padma Asana (Lotus Posture)

Parivritta Parshvakona (Turned Side-Angle Posture)

Paschimottan Asana (Posterior Stretching Pose)

Pavana Mukta Asana (Wind-Releasing Posture)

Sarvaung Asana (Shoulder Stand Posture)

Setu Bandhasana (Bridge Pose)

Shalabha Asana (Grasshopper Posture)

Shava Asana (Corspe Posture)

Siddha Asana (Straight Posture)

Simha Asana (Lion Posture)

Sirsha Asana (Headstand Posture)

Sukh Asana (Meditation Pose)

Tada Asana (Mountain Pose)

Trikona Asana (Triangle Pose)

Ushtra Asana (Camel Posture)

Urdhva Mukha Svan Asana (Up Dog Pose)

Utkat Asana (Chair Pose)

Virabhadr Asana I (Warrior I Pose)

Virabhadr Asana II (Warrior II Pose)

Virabhadr Asana III (Warrior III Pose)

Vira Asana (Hero Posture)

Vriksha Asana (Tree Pose)

Vrischika Asana (Scorpion Pose

Journal Entries

Journal Entry 1

This is my third semester in Melinda Smith's yoga class. The first semester was an eye opening, pure learning experience about yoga. I approached it with trepidation. My two great fears were my age, and muscular inflexibility. Namely, that I might not be able to keep up with the movements required, and that they were for younger persons. That fear dissipated quickly. It dissipated partly through the structure, patience, and insight of the instructor; and partly through my willingness to challenge my body in ways that I hadn't before. The flexibility concern was over the stiffness and lack of muscular flexibility from years of running.

I overcame that through the willingness to push my body (and mind).

The second semester the focus was on the meditative aspects of yoga. My focus was on concentration, relaxation, and freeing the mind, body, and spirit to prepare myself for a meditative experience that would truly free the mind of the mental baggage and clutter. The continuous positive affirmations from the instructor was and has been tantamount to a guided meditation session each class. It has been immensely instructive and guiding.

This semester I have chosen to place special emphasis on breathing. I have long been aware that breathing is the secret to focus, concentration, inner awareness, and attaining a true meditative state. But it's also something that has to be worked at and is not automatic. I am also aware that it's not necessary to completely control the breath which is not fully possible but to experience it and a focal point to fix awareness of self. There are several specific things I am working hard in an effort to master breathing as the entry point for meditative focus. One is to attain a consistent rhythm and harmony in my breathing.

The next is to draw mental energy and focus from the breathing. Another is to use the rhythm of my breathing to empty the mind of thoughts (clutter if you will) in order to attain mental openness and clarity. The final thing is to keep my focus on the inhaling and exhaling breaths. I am told that both are the two poles or forms of energy within our physical and subtle bodies and are the forces of positive and negative energy, the yin and yang, of our being.

The goal then this semester is to be continually aware of the importance of breathing in all of the yoga movements. That means incorporating breathing techniques in all of the yoga movements. It means using breathing as a focus and guide for opening my mind to positive, liberating thoughts and affirmations. Most importantly, it means using the body's most natural and life giving and affirming mechanism and this is breathing, to attain a true state of wellness and well-being.

Journal Entry 2

In my one year and a half yoga journey, I have focused on getting a handle on three areas. One is breathing, another is meditation. The third is muscular flexibility. I have certainly gained valued information, insight, and the practical application of techniques to enhance proper breathing and to attain a better balanced meditative state. Now for flexibility.

There were two challenges in using yoga techniques and postures to attain greater flexibility. The first challenge was age. The inescapable fact is that with the aging process there is flexibility loss. Obviously the average 60 year old can't move the muscles and joints as fluidly as a 20 year old. The second challenge was I have been a runner for many years. I have run 7 marathons and countless 5 and 10K races and I still run five days a week. Flexibility has always been a huge issue with runners—of any age. We just simply do not pay enough attention to prolonged and proper stretching before and after runs. Yoga was a partial antidote to that.

The yoga class sessions have placed a great deal of emphasis through the various postures on stretching the legs, neck, back, and stomach muscles out. But the area of greatest concern for me has been the leg muscles. The up and down dog positions, the warrior positions, and most importantly the leg flexors standing and prone have been of tremendous value to me. They have greatly improved my level and degree of flexibility.

The other stretch position (as well as meditative and for extending gratitude) is the heart opener. At the end of every run, I do a series of neck, back, and chest extensions—the heart opener. I give praise to God, life, and the universe for my life, my being, and the countless blessings of life bestowed on my family, friends, and all. I combine two things—the joy of the spirit and the joy of life in these stretching yoga postures.

The other byproduct of yoga stretches has been a reduced risk of injury from pulled and sore muscles. This has always been a major problem and concern of mine over the years and has accounted for numerous visits to my chiropractor.

Breathing, meditation, postures, spiritual well-being, and lastly flexibility have been the lasting rewarding returns from my years attempting to master the rudiments of yoga and incorporate them into my daily being. It's a work in progress and one I will continue to pursue in my life.

I'm deeply grateful that I've had the great fortune to have a phenomenal and supportive instructor. If nothing else in life, I've learned that having that kind of teacher is the indispensable ingredient to ultimate success in any every of study.

Much Thanks

Journal Entry 3

Book: Chinmoy, Sri, Yoga and the Spiritual life: The Journey of India's Soul (Aum Pubns; First edition (March 1, 1974)

1. Kapalbhati Pranayam: The Shining Forehead Breath

2. This is a simple, but effective method of doing two things to develop focus and concentration in breathing. It forces one to slow down the pace and repetition of breathing. This in turn forces the mind to focus exclusively on the inhalation and exhalation of breathing. The added beauty of this simple but effective breathing technique is that it strengthens the diaphragm and stomach muscles. The benefits then are both mental and physical.

3. I see no physical risks in this type of breathing

technique. In fact, the slow, methodical repetitive nature of this breathing virtually insures that this does not cause undue physical stress during the exhalation of the diaphragm.

4. I inhale as normal through the nostrils. I try to take in as much air as possible—filling up the lungs so to speak—and letting the abdomen expand. The exhalation is also through the nostrils but with a mild even exaggerated degree of force and making sure that I use my stomach muscles to aid in the exhalation (for added force). I repeat this as many times as I feel comfortable with. That's usually 10 to 12 minutes.

5. The time for the breath pose is 10 to 12 minutes. I prefer time to counting breaths. The count could be a distraction from my prime goal which is to use the breath as a tool to free the mind, and facilitate focus and concentration.

6. The one counter pose I have tried with limited success and patience is the breathing technique that stresses breathing through each nostril separately while covering the other nostril—Anulom Vilom Pranayam: Alternate Nostril Breath. This is not a comfortable technique for me primarily because I

must now concentrate on the separation of the breathing itself. By contrast, the other pose is simple and straightforward.

7. yogajournal.com, and wikihow

8. yoga citta vrtti nirodhaha

I like the conventional, literal meaning of this sutra. That is vritti means whirlpool. This is an appropriate definition and by extension this yoga sutra. Our minds are a continual whirlpool of ideas, thoughts, and reflections. Flowing from this mental turbulence are our doubts, worries, concerns, preoccupations, and stresses. The prime goal and challenge is how to "silence" or calm or even tame this whirlpool of mental turbulence. This is the key to engendering, or perhaps entering is a more accurate way of stating it, a heightened state of mental peace, tranquility, and harmony. According to the philosophy of this sutra, this is the direct pathway to attaining enlightenment about being, self, the world within and without.

Journal Entry 4

Interestingly, according to the wikipedia description of yoga citta vrtti nirodhaha, there is scientific evidence that found that this sutra actually stimulates the glands to secrete hormones (maybe endorphins) that aid in the attainment of a settled mental state.

abhysa vairagyabhyam tan nirodhah

Put simply this is the sutra that stresses practice, practice, practice to calm the mind, slow down the whirlpool, and agitation of our mental processes. This, of course, takes intense discipline, focus and concentration. Or put another way, one has to "detach" the mental turbulence of their thoughts. This again takes practice, practice, and more practice. It does not come natural. The metaphor that is used is that of a river and the need to give shape to its flow, rhythm, and release to awareness.

samtosad anuttamah sukhalabhah

Abraham Lincoln is reputed to have one said that "a person can be about as happy as they want to be." I thought of this Lincolnesque aphorism when reading about this sutra. Now Lincoln as far as we know never studied or practiced yoga. But he discovered the eternal truth of this sutra and that is one can attain true contentment by thinking, focusing on and embodying joyful thoughts. Turning doom and gloom on its head and find joy both within and without whether it's a walk in the park on a cool, breezy, but sunny day or simply looking for and discovering joy in our day to day relationships and life. Another way to put it is this perception becomes reality. If we think joy and contentment constantly we will find it and attain it.

Finally, it means acceptance of those things that can't be changed, and changing those things that can. First and foremost that means our thoughts, perceptions, and being.

Journal Entry 5

The time for the breath pose is 10 to 12 minutes. I prefer time to counting breaths. The count could be a distraction from my prime goal which is to use the breath as a tool to free the mind, and facilitate focus and concentration.

I practiced the breathing techniques minimum five minutes on these dates:

June 16, 2017

June 18, 2017

June 20, 2017

June 22, 2017

June 24, 2017

June 26, 2017

June 28, 2017

July 1, 2017

July 3, 2017

July 5, 2017

July 7, 2017

July 9, 2017

July 11, 2017

July 13, 2017

and every other subsequent day in July 2017

Notes

Introduction

Fitness Magazine Editors, "Yoga Poses for Beginners," https://www.fitnessmagazine.com/workout/yoga/poses/beginner-yoga-poses/, ND

Mercer, Lisa, "Controversy on the Benefits of Yoga," Arizona Central, http://healthyliving.azcentral.com/controversy-benefits-yoga-12776.html ND

1—A Walk through Yoga's Past

https://en.wikipedia.org/wiki/Asana

Carrico, Mara, "Get to Know the Eight Limbs of Yoga," August 28, 2007, https://www.yogajournal.com/practice/the-eight-limbs#!

Chinmoy, Sri, *Yoga and the Spiritual life: The Journey of India's Soul* (Haldwani, India: Aum Publications, March 1, 1974)

Yogi Ramacharaka, *Raja Yoga or Mental Development: A Series of Lessons* (Chicago: Yogi Publication Society, 1934)

Carrico, Mara, "A Beginner's Guide to the History of Yoga, Where it all began—learn about the history of yoga, the roots of this ancient practice," https://www.yogajournal.com/yoga-101/the-roots-of-yoga#!, August 28, 2007

"History of Yoga: How it all Started," https://yoga.com/article/history-of-yoga-how-it-all-started, ND

2—Take a Yoga Break

http://yogadork.com/2013/06/17/yoga-related-studies-are-increasing/

http://www.med-health.net/5-Health-Problems-That-Yoga-Is-an-Answer-To.html

http://www.webmd.com/balance/news/20131230/what-yoga-can-and-cant-do-for-you#3

Park, Justin "The Truth About 7 Big Yoga Claims, Which promises can your practice truly deliver on?, http://www.shape.com/fitness/tips/truth-about-7-big-yoga-claims, ND

Broad, William, The Healing Power of Yoga Controversy," *New York Times,* January 10, 2013

3—Fact and Fiction About Yoga

https://www.washingtonpost.com/opinions/five-myths-about-yoga/2015/08/14/2b4c8638-41ce-11e5-846d-02792f854297_story.html?utm_term=.db37593c761c

Gabbert, Cheryl, "Yoga For the Not-So Spiritually Minded," http://www.healthguideinfo.com/yoga-and-pilates-articles/p22779/, May 16, 2011

http://www.healthguideinfo.com/yoga-and-pilates-articles/p22779/

Pizer, Ann, "Most Popular Types of Yoga Explained, Summary of the Most Popular Types of Contemporary Yoga," https://www.verywell.com/types-of-yoga-cheat-sheet-3566894, April 26, 2017

Gregoire, Carolyn, "How Yoga Became A $27 Billion Industry—And Reinvented American Spirituality," http://www.huffingtonpost.com/2013/12/16/how-the-yoga-industry-los_n_4441767.html, December 16, 2013

Moran, Susan, "Meditate on This: Yoga Is Big Business," http://www.nytimes.com/2006/12/28/business/28sbiz.html, December 28, 2006

William J. Broad, *The Science of Yoga: The Risks and Rewards,* (New York: Simon & Schuster, 2012)

4—America's Rush to the Mat

NIH, "Americans who practice Yoga report better wellness, health behaviors," https://www.nih.gov/news-events/news-releases/americans-who-practice-yoga-report-better-wellness-health-behaviors, November 4, 2015

https://www.usatoday.com/story/news/nation/2015/03/01/yoga-health-fitness-trends/23881391/

https://www.cnbc.com/2014/08/25/yoga-on-wall-street-big-time-bankers-seek-edge-on-the-yoga-mat.html

Miller, Korin, "Why Doctors Are Endorsing Yoga Instead of Opioids for Lower Back Pain," https://www.yahoo.com/beauty/why-doctors-endorsing-yoga-instead-191750073.html, February 15, 2017

5—Only the Mat Was Black

Lawrence, Stewart, "Is American Yoga Racist,"

https://www.counterpunch.org/2013/10/28/is-american-yoga-racist, October 28, 2013

https://www.forbes.com/sites/alicegwalton/2014/08/14/on-yogas-race-problem-has-the-practice-become-too-white/#26141f706ddb, October 28, 2013

http://yogadork.com/2015/05/21/the-struggle-of-the-black-yogi/

Daya Devi-Doolin, *Yoga, Meditation and Spiritual Growth for the African American Community: If You Can Breathe You Can Do Yoga and Find Inner and Outer Peace* (Phoenix, Ariz.: Amber Communications Group, 2014)

6—Where are the Guys?

http://www.yogamartusa.com/Yoga_Lowdown-Why-are-not-more-men-in-Yoga-class.html

https://www.washingtonpost.com/national/health-science/why-yoga-is-still-dominated-by-women-despite-the-medical-benefits-to-both-sexes/2013/10/21/a924bed2-34f5-11e3-80c6-7e6dd8d22d8f_story.html?utm_term=.73489a36d0d7

Broad, William J., *The Science of Yoga: The Risks*

and the Rewards (New York: Simon & Schuster)

https://www.cheatsheet.com/health-fitness/why-more-men-should-be-doing-yoga.html/?a=viewall

Testing Pohlman, "Stop Trying to Make Men Do Yoga," http://manflowyoga.com/blog/stop-trying-to-make-men-do-yoga/, January 23, 2014

https://www.nytimes.com/2015/08/30/sports/football/players-turning-to-yoga-as-a-way-to-stay-in-shape.html

http://nflfilms.nfl.com/2013/06/21/behind-the-scenes-yoga-and-football/

Costa, Chloe Della, "Why More Men Should be Doing Yoga," http://www.mensfitness.com/training/pro-tips/9-reasons-why-you-should-practice-yoga, March 23, 2016

Conclusion—The State of Yoga and Me

www.yogajournal.com/yogainamericastudy and www.yogaalliance.org/2016yogainamericastudy.

New Yoga Demographic Survey from Yoga Alliance https://www.yogaalliance.org/Learn/Article_Archive/Wakefield_Yoga_Survey, June 18, 2015

About the Author

Earl Ofari Hutchinson is a nationally known political analyst and author of books on race and politics. He is an associate editor of New America Media. He is a weekly co-host of the *Al Sharpton Show* on Radio One. He is the host of the weekly *Hutchinson Report* on KPFK 90.7 FM Los Angeles and the Pacifica Network.

He has been a practitioner of yoga for years. He has learned, trained, and studied yoga practices, techniques and philosophy under four of Southern California's leading yoga instructors at Body and Brain Studios in Los Angeles and West Los Angeles College. He has interviewed and discussed yoga practices and the yoga industry on his Pacifica Radio Show, The Hutchinson Report.

www.ingramcontent.com/pod-product-compliance
Lightning Source LLC
Chambersburg PA
CBHW072101040426
42334CB00041B/1874